50 Studies Every Global Health Provider Should Know

50 STUDIES EVERY DOCTOR SHOULD KNOW

50 Studies Every Doctor Should Know: The Key Studies That Form the Foundation of Evidence Based Medicine, Revised Edition
Michael E. Hochman

50 Studies Every Internist Should Know
Kristopher Swiger, Joshua R. Thomas, Michael E. Hochman, and Steven Hochman

50 Studies Every Neurologist Should Know
David Y. Hwang and David M. Greer

50 Studies Every Pediatrician Should Know
Ashaunta T. Anderson, Nina L. Shapiro, Stephen C. Aronoff, Jeremiah Davis, and Michael Levy

50 Imaging Studies Every Doctor Should Know
Christoph I. Lee

50 Studies Every Surgeon Should Know
SreyRam Kuy, Rachel J. Kwon, and Miguel A. Burch

50 Studies Every Intensivist Should Know
Edward A. Bittner

50 Studies Every Palliative Care Doctor Should Know
David Hui, Akhila Reddy, and Eduardo Bruera

50 Studies Every Psychiatrist Should Know
Ish P. Bhalla, Rajesh R. Tampi, and Vinod H. Srihari

50 Studies Every Anesthesiologist Should Know
Anita Gupta, Michael E. Hochman, and Elena N. Gutman

50 Studies Every Ophthalmologist Should Know
Alan D. Penman, Kimberly W. Crowder, and William M. Watkins, Jr.

50 Studies Every Urologist Should Know
Philipp Dahm

50 Studies Every Obstetrician and Gynecologist Should Know
Constance Liu, Noah Rindos, and Scott Shainker

50 Studies Every Doctor Should Know: The Key Studies That Form the Foundation of Evidence-Based Medicine, 2nd Edition
Michael E. Hochman and Steven D. Hochman

50 Studies Every Occupational Therapist Should Know
Elizabeth A. Pyatak and Elissa S. Lee

50 Studies Every Vascular Surgeon Should Know
Julien Al Shakarchi

50 Studies Every Global Health Provider Should Know
Andrea Walker, Anup Agarwal, and Yogesh Jain

50 Studies Every Global Health Provider Should Know

EDITED BY

ANDREA WALKER, ANUP AGARWAL, AND YOGESH JAIN

SERIES EDITOR

MICHAEL E. HOCHMAN

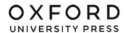

OXFORD
UNIVERSITY PRESS

Oxford University Press is a department of the University of Oxford. It furthers
the University's objective of excellence in research, scholarship, and education
by publishing worldwide. Oxford is a registered trade mark of Oxford University
Press in the UK and certain other countries.

Published in the United States of America by Oxford University Press
198 Madison Avenue, New York, NY 10016, United States of America.

Library of Congress Cataloging-in-Publication Data
Names: Walker, Andrea, editor. | Agarwal, Anup, MBBS, editor. | Jain, Yogesh, editor.
Title: 50 studies every global health provider should know /
edited by Andrea Walker, Anup Agarwal, Yogesh Jain.
Other titles: Fifty studies every global health provider should know |
50 studies every doctor should know (Series)
Description: New York, NY : Oxford University Press, [2023] |
Series: 50 studies every doctor should know | Includes bibliographical references and index.
Identifiers: LCCN 2023003840 (print) | LCCN 2023003841 (ebook) |
ISBN 9780197548721 (paperback) | ISBN 9780197548745 (epub) | ISBN 9780197548752
Subjects: MESH: Global Health | Developing Countries | Vulnerable Populations
Classification: LCC RA441 (print) | LCC RA441 (ebook) | NLM WA 530.1 |
DDC 362.1—dc23/eng/20230429
LC record available at https://lccn.loc.gov/2023003840
LC ebook record available at https://lccn.loc.gov/2023003841

DOI: 10.1093/med/9780197548721.001.0001

This material is not intended to be, and should not be considered, a substitute for medical or other
professional advice. Treatment for the conditions described in this material is highly dependent on the
individual circumstances. And, while this material is designed to offer accurate information with respect
to the subject matter covered and to be current as of the time it was written, research and knowledge about
medical and health issues is constantly evolving and dose schedules for medications are being revised
continually, with new side effects recognized and accounted for regularly. Readers must therefore always
check the product information and clinical procedures with the most up-to-date published product
information and data sheets provided by the manufacturers and the most recent codes of conduct and safety
regulation. The publisher and the authors make no representations or warranties to readers, express or
implied, as to the accuracy or completeness of this material. Without limiting the foregoing, the publisher
and the authors make no representations or warranties as to the accuracy or efficacy of the drug dosages
mentioned in the material. The authors and the publisher do not accept, and expressly disclaim, any
responsibility for any liability, loss, or risk that may be claimed or incurred as a consequence of the use and/or
application of any of the contents of this material.

Printed by Sheridan Books, Inc., United States of America

CONTENTS

SECTION 4 Child Health

SECTION 5 Women's Health

SECTION 6 Mental Health

SECTION 7 Noncommunicable Diseases

SECTION 8 Surgery

CONTRIBUTORS

Anup Agarwal, MBBS
Academic Hospitalist
Medstar Health Baltimore
Baltimore, MD, USA
Assistant Professor
Georgetown University School of
    Medicine
Washington, DC, USA

Anurima Baidya, MBBS, MPH
Research Associate
Department of International Health
Johns Hopkins Bloomberg School of
    Public Health
Baltimore, MD, USA

Jessica Bender, MD, MPH
Clinical Assistant Professor
Division of General Internal Medicine
University of Washington
Seattle, WA, USA

Amanda Bradke, MD
Assistant Professor
Department of Internal Medicine
Rush University Medical Center
Chicago, IL, USA

Cristina Rivera Carpenter, PhD
Navajo Nation Program Officer,
    HEAL Initiative
University of California
Sanfrancisco, CA, USA

Riti Chandrashekhar, MHS
Research Assistant
Johns Hopkins University
Baltimore, MD, USA

Pranab Chatterjee, MD
PhD Candidate
Department of International Health
Johns Hopkins Bloomberg School of
    Public Health
Baltimore, MD, USA

**Shaheen Chowdhury, DNB
(Family Medicine)**
Internal Medicine Resident
Cambridge Health Alliance
Boston, MA, USA

Georgery Constant, MD
Zanmi Lasante/Partners in Health
Cange, Haiti

Nadra Crawford, MD, MPH
Family Medicine Physician
Zuni Comprehensive Community
    Health Center
Zuni, NM, USA

Nakyda Dean, MD
HEAL Initiative Fellow
University of California
San Francisco, CA, USA

**Jack Fukushima, Medical Student,
MD/PhD Candidate**
UCLA David Geffen School of
    Medicine
Los Angeles, CA, USA

**Anita Gadgil, MBBS, MS, DNB
(Gen. Surgery)**
Head, Department of Surgery
Bhabha Atomic Research Centre
    (BARC) Hospital
Mumbai, India
WHO Collaboration Centre for
    Research in Surgical Care Delivery
    in LMICs
Mumbai, MH, India

Tushar Garg, MBBS, MPH
Postdoctoral Fellow
Department of Epidemiology
Johns Hopkins Bloomberg School of
    Public Health
Baltimore, MD, USA

Bassem Ghali, MD
Assistant Professor
Department of Medicine
University of California
San Francisco, CA, USA

Robin Goldman, MD, MPH
Associate Professor
San Francisco VA Medical Center
    University of California
San Francisco, CA, USA

**Arkaprabha Gun, Master of Arts
(M.A.) in Economics**
Research Associate
International AIDS Vaccine Initiative
Delhi, India

**Sadoscar Hakizimana, MD, MMED,
FCOG(ECSA)**
Master of Medical Science in Global
    Health Delivery
Harvard Medical School/Partners in
    Health
Boston, MA, USA

Kuang-Ning Huang, MD
Department of Family Medicine
University of Washington
Seattle, WA, USA

Priyank Jain, MBBS
Department of Internal Medicine,
    Cambridge Health Alliance
Assistant Professor of Medicine
Harvard Medical School
Boston, MA, USA

E. John Ly, MD
Medical Director
Last Mile Health, Monrovia, Liberia
Associate Program Director
Med-Peds residency
David Geffen School of Medicine at
    University of California
Los Angeles, CA, USA

Arnold Jumbe, MD, MBA
Director of Health and Social Services
Thyolo District Council
Thyolo, Southern Region, Malawi

Sitalire Kapira, MD
Master of Medical Science in Global
 Health Delivery
Harvard Medical School
Boston, USA
Maternal and Child Health Specialist
 Partners In Health
Blantyre, Malawi

Colleen Keough, MD, MPH
Assistant Professor
Internal Medicine and Pediatrics
Baylor College of Medicine
Houston, TX, USA

Abhisake Kole, MD, PhD
Department of Medicine
Emory University
Atlanta, GA, USA

Timothy S. Laux, MD, MPH
Hospitalist
Cambridge Health Alliance
Cambridge, MA, USA

Alexa Lindley, MD, MPH
Department of Family Medicine
University of Washington
Seattle, WA, USA

Rodrigo Bazua Lobato, MD
PhD Candidate
Harvard T.H. Chan School of
 Public Health
Boston, MA, USA

Rachel Lusk, MD
Assistant Professor at the University
 of Arizona
Pediatrics
District Medical Group / Valleywise
 Health
Phoenix, AZ, USA

Monali Mohan, MBBS
Consultant
WHO Collaboration Centre for
 Research in Surgical Care Delivery
 in LMICs
Mumbai, MH, India

Rose L. Molina, MD, MPH
Assistant Professor of Obstetrics
Gynecology and Reproductive
 Biology
Department of Obstetrics and
 Gynecology
Beth Israel Deaconess Medical Center
Boston, MA, USA

Mariana Montano, MD
Compañeros En Salud
Calle Primera Poniente
Ángel Albino Corzo, Chiapas, Mexico

Peter Olds, MD, MPH
Instructor in Medicine
Massachusetts General Hospital
Boston, MA, USA
Harvard Medical School
Boston, MA, USA

Maria Openshaw, MS, CNM
Assistant Clinical Professor
University of California
San Francisco School of Nursing
San Francisco, CA, USA

Jessica C. Parker, DO
Pediatric Emergency Medicine Fellow
Children's Mercy Kansas City
Kansas City, MO, USA

Shyamsundar J. Raithatha, MD
Community Physician
Tribal Integrated Development
  and Education (TIDE)
  Trustshali Trust
Gujarat, India

**Nobhojit Roy, MBBS, MS
(Gen. Surgery), MPH, PhD**
Public Health Systems
Karolinska Institute
Stockholm, Sweden
WHO Collaboration Centre for
  Research in Surgical Care Delivery
  in LMICs
Mumbai, MH, India

Vidiya Sathananthan, MD
Jackson Memorial Hospital/
  University of Miami
Miami, FL, USA

Casey Sautter, MD
HEAL Initiative Fellow
University of California
San Francisco, CA, USA

Trisha Schimek, MD, MPH
Department of Family Medicine
Contra Costa Regional Medical Center
Martinez, CA, USA

Bhavna Seth, MD, MHS
Pulmonary Critical Care Fellow
Johns Hopkins University
Baltimore, MD, USA

Naman Shah, MD, PhD
Family Medicine Physician
Los Angeles, CA, USA

Priyansh Shah, MBBS
Intern Doctor
Baroda Medical College
Vadodara, India
President
World Youth Heart Federation
Vadodara, India
WHO Collaboration Centre for
  Research in Surgical Care Delivery
  in LMICs
Mumbai, MH, India

Ryan Shields, MD
Obstetrics/Gynencology
Gallup Indian Medical Center
Gallup, NM, USA

Linda Shipton, MD
Assistant Professor of Medicine
Harvard Medical School
Infectious Disease Specialist
  Cambridge Health Alliance
Cambridge, MA, USA

Shegufta Shefa Sikder, PhD
Global Disease Control & Epidemiology
Senior Technical Advisor at CARE USA
Washington, DC, USA

Stephanie Sirna, MD
Assistant Professor of Medicine
Department of Medicine
Weill Cornell Medical College
New York, NY, USA

Erica Tate, MD
Section of General Internal
  Medicine & Geriatrics
Associate Program Director
Internal Medicine
John W. Deming Department of
  Medicine
Tulane University School of Medicine
New Orleans, LA, USA

Jessica Top, MD
Pediatrics
University of South Dakota Sanford
    School of Medicine
Sioux Falls, SD, USA

Frances Ue, MD, MPH
Department of Medicine
Cambridge Health Alliance, Harvard
    Medical School Cambridge
MA, USA

Andrea Walker, MD
Obestetrics and Gynecology
Gallup Community Health
Gallup, NM, USA

Ami Waters, MD, MPH
Department of Pediatrics
University of Texas Southwestern
Dallas, Texas, USA
Last Mile Health, Monrovia, Liberia

Jennifer Werdenberg, MD, MPH
Assistant Professor
Baylor College of Medicine
Houston, Texas, USA
Pediatric Hospitalist
Texas Children's Hospital
Houston, Texas, USA

Rebecca White, MD
Department of Psychiatry
Western Michigan University
    Homer Stryker M.D. School of
    Medicine
Kalamazoo, MI, USA

Lena Wong, MD, MPH
Fellow in Infectious Disease
University of Miami/Jackson
    Memorial Hospital
Miami, FL, USA

INTRODUCTION

Health is a fundamental human right, but discrepancies in health outcomes exist globally—between high-income countries and low-income countries, and between marginalized groups within both. Our purpose in writing *50 Studies Every Global Health Provider Should Know* is to recognize and summarize studies that have transnational implications for healthcare among marginalized populations due to geographic, cultural, or socioeconomic reasons. Our goal is to provide readers with information that can be built upon and utilized in their own healthcare contexts to narrow the healthcare discrepancy gap, as well as to encourage advocacy and collaboration.

There are many definitions of "global health." Since no term better identifies the field of healthcare providers interested in health equity, we entitled this book *50 Studies Every Global Health Provider Should Know*, while recognizing the limitations of the expression "global health." This term is broad and is used largely in parts of North America and Europe, with minimal use in Africa, Asia, and Latin America. It has multiple connotations, ranging from colonial health, social medicine, and health equity. One of the most crucial overtones of global health is in defining and characterizing the power differential between the provider (funder, healthcare provider, or policymaker, usually based in high-income countries) and the provided (usually marginalized populations). However, it also includes a focus on social justice as it endeavors to identify social forces and policies that underlie the ailments of a population. Other aspects of global health range from program planning and healthcare delivery in resource-limited settings, to the pathologies more prevalent among marginalized groups. Recognizing these limitations, we decided on the term "global health" to underline the importance of healthcare as a fundamental human right and the goal to address healthcare disparities globally.

Choosing 50 studies was challenging given that the field of global health is unique in that it is a broad field that covers an extensive range of topics and thus requires the inclusion of nonclinical phenomena that affect health outcomes. We first chose the eight major sections of the book: Health Systems and Healthcare Delivery, Social Medicine and Ethics, Infectious Diseases and Neglected Tropical Diseases, Child Health, Women's Health, Mental Health, Noncommunicable Diseases, and Surgery. Within these sections, we searched for seminal publications such as systematic reviews, reports from multilateral agencies, and reports from international consensus-building efforts, such as the Lancet Commissions and experts in the field. However, this still did not give us the number or variety of studies we sought for each section.

While choosing the studies for inclusion in the book, all three editors were working in rural and underserved parts of Liberia, the United States, Malawi, and India. In order to gain the diversity in studies we were aiming for, we began to look critically into our daily work and examined the evidence behind the interventions that our colleagues, organizations, or partners in the respective ministries of health were using. This examination formed the conceptual foundation for the identification of the 50 studies in this book. This book includes many landmark studies which were subsequently translated into guidelines that affect practice globally, making this a practice-informed effort.

Moreover, global health is inherently political, and so we conceptualized this work to be not merely a technical commentary, but a social one. As you read through the book, we hope you will gain insight into a variety of perspectives, political and social analyses, and implementation efforts surrounding public and global health research. Some critical topics not explored in this book include refugee and incarcerated populations, substance use, palliative care, historical trauma, colonialism, and climate change and its impact on health. This is largely because much of the research or discourse surrounding these topics is written in formats that are not conducive to the study design best utilized by the format of this book series. We accept this as a significant limitation of this volume.

Most books on global health are written by authors whose major affiliations and work are in the Global North. We attempted to mitigate this in both the choice of studies for inclusion as well as in the selection of chapter authors. Where multiple articles may illustrate similar conclusions, we prioritized equity by choosing articles authored by members of underrepresented populations. We ensured that chapter authors had significant experience working with underserved populations and invited authors from a variety of healthcare disciplines, including nurses, midwives, public health specialists, epidemiologists, economists, physicians, and clinical officers. This led to a diverse mix of authors from seven countries, which we feel is the most vital asset of this undertaking.

We recognize that an academic exercise such as writing this book is a privilege afforded to few practitioners working with marginalized people. Most practitioners in resource-denied settings find it challenging to remain updated with scientific literature because of busy schedules, difficult work conditions, the high cost of journal subscriptions, and a lack of institutional support for education. This book can serve as a primer for providers in such communities to understand and examine the literature behind the healthcare interventions they provide. While researching, we reviewed our own biases: Directly Observed Therapy short-course (DOTS) in TB, training and supervision in maternal health, or steroids in meningitis. Similarly, we hope every reader will be able to reflect critically on their work and eventually work toward building evidence.

About the Sections and Studies

For Section 1, Health Systems and Healthcare Delivery, we chose studies that underline the importance of a community-based approach, community health workers, informal providers, and primary healthcare facility interventions. We especially emphasize the important role of community health workers in designing health systems, and we have included nine studies that highlight the role of community health workers in delivering care for multi-drug-resistant tuberculosis (TB), home-based neonatal care, integrated management of childhood illnesses, and managing noncommunicable diseases using mobile health technology.

Martin Luther King Jr. remarked: "Of all the forms of inequality, injustice in healthcare is the most shocking and the most inhumane." Section 2, Social Medicine and Ethics—arguably the most important section in this book and a worthy read as an entire book on its own—takes care to include studies demonstrating injustice in healthcare and the impact of socioeconomic class, gender, nutrition, race, and power in the health of populations. This section includes landmark studies that help form the basis of the argument for the social determinants of health, including the Barker Hypothesis, Whitehall studies, and the Papworth experiment.

In Section 3, Infectious and Neglected Tropical Diseases, we chose to focus on HIV, TB, malaria, diarrhea, pneumonia, and COVID-19. We selected studies on pre-exposure chemoprophylaxis for HIV, prevention of mother-to-child transmission of HIV through breastfeeding, and optimal timing for initiation of HIV treatment. Similarly, for TB, we chose studies that highlight the importance of household contact investigation, prevention of TB, and treatment for multi-drug-resistant TB. For malaria, we chose a landmark study on prevention using insecticide-treated bed nets and another examining the importance of artesunate in treatment of malaria. We included the SOLIDARITY trial, as it was one of the most extensive adaptive trials on COVID-19 initiated by the World Health Organization (WHO) and provides a model to follow for future global collaborative effort. Finally, we included a study on the use of steroids in meningitis to demonstrate that the efficacy of similar drug regimens may differ depending on health systems and patient populations.

Five studies were included in Section 4 on Child Health, though there is considerable overlap with other sections. As diarrheal illness is a major cause of morbidity and mortality in children worldwide, we included a study on zinc and diarrhea. Similarly, Helping Babies Breathe has been widely implemented at births. Bubble CPAP (continuous positive airway pressure) is one of the most common lifesaving strategies in pediatric intensive care units globally. We included the use of hydroxyurea in sickle cell disease because it is a life-altering intervention and highlights the population that suffers from this disease. The FEAST trial stresses, again, the fact that similar interventions may have varied outcomes depending on the clinical context.

Our study selection in Section 5, Women's Health, mirrors the skew of research in resource-denied settings toward obstetrical issues rather than gynecologic issues. Four of the five chapters in this section are associated with maternal health, including aspirin in pregnancy for the prevention of preeclampsia, magnesium sulfate for the prevention of seizures in preeclampsia, tranexamic acid to treat postpartum hemorrhage, and the use of partograms in labor rooms to enable early and effective labor intervention. Visual inspection with acetic acid for cervical cancer screening was included, as this is often utilized in resource-denied settings instead of pap smear or HPV (human papillomavirus) testing to screen for a leading cause of cancer death in women globally that can be cured early with effective screening and treatment methods. There is some overlap with other sections again here, as we include a study on syndromic management of STDs in the infectious disease section. Notably absent is breast cancer screening, heavy menstrual bleeding, contraception, HPV vaccination, and abortion care. This is largely due to a paucity of studies applicable in low-resource settings or a lack of translation of research into practice.

In Section 6, Mental Health, we have included three studies highlighting the importance of primary care and community-based interventions in managing mental health in low-resource settings. These studies overlap with the Health Systems and Healthcare Delivery section, but they were separated to highlight the importance of mental health, which is often neglected and underfunded globally.

Although the burden of Noncommunicable Diseases (NCDs) is rising globally, Section 7 includes only three studies largely because NCD treatment is still an aspiration in many parts of the world. We have included one study on the use of aspirin in stroke as that is the most commonly available treatment, and one study on use Streptokinase in Acute myocardial infarction as cardiac catheterization is inaccessible in most parts of the world. Lastly, we have also included the SPRINT trial. As the management of hypertension is not generally resource-intensive, this chapter is meant to emphasize the importance of context in health-care provision and how to responsibly adapt research from resource-abundant settings to resource-constrained settings.

Section 8, Global Surgery, incorporates three studies that focus on lifesaving measures in the field. Ketamine is a commonly used deep-sedation anesthetic that is useful when general anesthesia is not available to perform lifesaving procedures. Task shifting for C-sections, one of the most critical lifesaving surgeries, is a common approach to improving patient access to care. Surgical checklists are low-cost interventions recommended by the WHO and are proven to reduce surgical morbidity and mortality.

Now that the rationale and heart behind the book have been explained, we expect that this work will provoke reflection in our daily interventions, the way social institutions affect our patients, and what we can do to narrow the health-care gap.

Andrea Walker—Obstetrics and Gynecology, Gallup Community Health, Gallup, NM, USA

Anup Agarwal—Academic Hospitalist, Medstar Health Baltimore, USA
Assistant Professor, Georgetown University School of Medicine, USA

Yogesh Jain—Public Health Physician, Chhattisgarh, India

Health Systems and Healthcare Delivery

For Section 1, Health Systems and Healthcare Delivery, we chose studies that underline the importance of a community-based approach, community health workers, informal providers, and primary healthcare facility interventions. We especially emphasize the important role of community health workers in designing health systems, and we have included nine studies that highlight the role of community health workers in delivering care for multi-drug-resistant tuberculosis (TB), home-based neonatal care, integrated management of childhood illnesses, and managing noncommunicable diseases using mobile health technology.

1

The Rwandan Experience

The Impact of Health Systems Strengthening Interventions in the Context of Prioritizing Health Equity

E. JOHN LY

> Our results show that historically unprecedented improvement in health indicators . . . is possible among its poorest and most geographically isolated residents. Notably, almost all of the decline in under-five mortality occurred among the lowest two wealth quintiles . . . where the intervention included specific components (subsidies of insurance premiums and copays, nutrition support and compensated village-based community health workers) designed to address inequities in access to care.
>
> RWANDA PHIT PARTNERSHIP[1,2]

Research Question: What is the role for carrying out multiple, integrated health systems strengthening interventions in improving population health coverage and outcomes?

Funding: Doris Duke Charitable Foundation's African Health Initiative

Year Study Began: 2005

Year Study Published: 2018

Study Location: Two rural districts in Rwanda (Kirehe, Southern Kayonza)

Who Was Studied: Women of reproductive age (15–49 years old), surveyed via Rwanda Demographic and Health Survey

Who Was Excluded: None

How Many Patients: 21,338

Study Overview: See Figure 1.1.

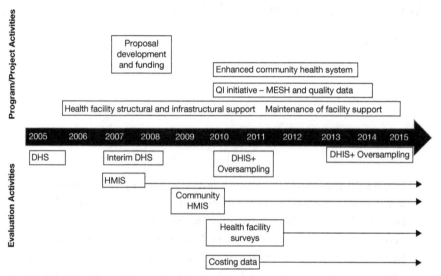

Figure 1.1. Overview of the study design.

Study Intervention: The Population Health Implementation and Training (PHIT) study investigators, a partnership including the Rwandan Ministry of Health and Partners in Health, worked together to implement health systems strengthening interventions in the southeastern region of Rwanda, that included Kirehe and S. Kiyonza. The interventions were focused around the WHO's six core health system building blocks.[3]

The six building blocks are:

- Service delivery
- Health workforce
- Health information systems
- Access to essential medicines
- Financing
- Leadership.

They were centered around targeted support to health facilities (including infrastructure improvement), quality improvement initiatives, and strengthening the network of community health workers. The comparison group was a composite of other rural areas of Rwanda, which were also seeing development support through Rwanda's Vision 2020 plan. The broader national program included a national health insurance scheme, a system of performance-based financing, and the expansion of a community health worker network.

Follow-Up: 10 years

Endpoints: The primary output indicators were assessed via the Rwanda Demographic Health Survey (RDHS).
Process indicators measure activities and outputs of the program, such as:

- Whether children under 5 years old received treatment for recent episodes of acute respiratory infection (ARI), diarrhea, or fever
- Whether children under 2 years old received a third dose of diphtheria-pertussispolio-tetanus (DPT) or measles vaccine

Outcome indicators measure end outcome-related expected changes from the program, such as:

- Neonatal mortality
- Adult mortality
- Recent occurrence of ARI, diarrhea, or fever in children under 5 years old.

RESULTS

Between 2005 and 2010:

- Health system coverage (as measured by a composite score of child health interventions) improved similarly from 57.9% to 75.0% in the intervention area and from 58.7% to 73.5% in other rural areas.
- Under-5 mortality decreased by an annual rate of 12.8% in the intervention area, and 8.9% in other rural areas. These trends were not significantly different between the two groups.
- The proportion of children treated for ARI rose from 18.7% to 54.6% in the intervention area and from 26.2% to 36.5% in other rural areas, which

was statistically significant. The trends adjusted for mother's age and household wealth were statistically significant for ARI, diarrhea, and fever in the intervention areas (Table 1.1).

- No other trends were statistically significant as improvements were seen in both intervention and non-intervention areas.

Table 1.1 SUMMARY OF KEY FINDINGS

Indicator	Region	2005	2010	Change (2005 vs. 2010)	p Value
Received measles vaccine (12–23 mo)	K/SK[a]	73.91%	92.08%	17.76	0.007
	ORA (control)[b]	85.59%	95.03%	9.02	<0.001
Vitamin A supplement in last 6 months (0–59 mo)	K/SK	77.27%	89.14%	11.70	<0.001
	ORA (control)	84.31%	93.07%	8.59	<0.001
ARI in last 2 weeks and received treatment (<5 yo)	K/SK	18.69%	54.58%	34.53	<0.001
	ORA (control)	26.19%	36.53%	8.97	0.001
Diarrhea in last 2 weeks and received ORT (<5 yo)	K/SK	12.12%	34.58%	21.22	0.003
	ORA (control)	17.74%	33.94%	14.97	<0.001
4+ antenatal visit (births last 5 years)	K/SK	10.35%	26.94%	16.05	<0.001
	ORA (control)	12.79%	35.22%	21.89	<0.001
Attended by a skilled health worker (births last 5 years)	K/SK	38.74%	64.48%	23.68	<0.001
	ORA (control)	34.37%	67.55%	31.12	<0.001
Current use of modern contraceptive (married women)	K/SK	13.85%	46.15%	29.67	<0.001
	ORA (control)	8.24%	44.79%	33.92	<0.001
Modified composite coverage index	K/SK	57.9	75.0	—	—
	ORA (control)	58.7	73.8	—	—
Under-5 mortality rate (per 1000 live birth)	K/SK	229.8	83.2	−146.6	<0.001
	ORA (control)	157.7	75.8	−81.9	<0.001

[a] Kirehe; Southern Kayonza
[b] Other rural areas.

Criticisms and Limitations:

The study was dependent on the Rwanda Demographic and Health Survey (RDHS) questions and responses from women, with findings subject to recall bias. While survey tools were selected to assess for health system coverage (availability of services), they were not designed to assess for the quality of care provided (such as the appropriateness of those services).

Other Relevant Studies and Information:

- The BetterBirth Trial group study demonstrated in a matched-pair, cluster-randomized, control trial in Uttar Pradesh, India, that coaching-based implementation of the WHO Safe Childbirth Checklist increased birth attendant adherence for 18 essential birth practices (72.8% vs. 41.2%, at 2 months) and (61.7% vs. 43.9% at 12 months), at intervention vs. control facilities, but did not lead to a significant difference in primary outcomes including perinatal or maternal death.[4]
- The Saving Mothers Giving Life program, a multi-partner effort, employed a districtwide health system strengthening approach in Uganda and Zambia and demonstrated a decline in maternal mortality by ~40% over 5 years. Their interventions addressed both supply- and demand-side interventions to ensure timely use of maternity health services.[5]

Summary and Implications: This analysis assessing the Population Health Implementation and Training team's work in Rwanda demonstrated substantial gains in health system coverage (there was an improvement from 57.9% to 75% in composite score for childhood health interventions) and in outcomes (12.8% annual reduction in childhood mortality), over 5 years from 2005 to 2010. This work demonstrates that multifaceted interventions aimed at strengthening health systems can improve population health outcomes.

CLINICAL CASE: ADDRESSING CHILDHOOD MORTALITY IN A HEALTH DISTRICT

Case History
A rural district in a resource-constrained country has been suffering from high rates of childhood mortality for many decades. A new district health team has

funding to reduce childhood deaths. They could choose to purchase medicines and supplies or work solely at the facility, or in the community. According to the findings of the Population Health Implementation and Training study in Rwanda, how should they proceed?

Suggested Answer

The PHIT study in Rwanda demonstrated that multiple interventions, addressing the following 6 core pillars of health systems, can be effective in achieving reductions in childhood mortality:

1. Service delivery
2. Health workforce
3. Information systems
4. Medical products and technology
5. Leadership and governance
6. Financing.

This health district team should plan a broad-based effort that includes community health, the facility, and general health system strengthening interventions. Rather than choosing an approach which is "either/or," the approach should be to strengthen every aspect of the 6 pillars of health systems.

References

1. Thomson DR, Amoroso C, Atwood S, et al. Impact of a health system strengthening intervention on maternal and child health outputs and outcomes in rural Rwanda 2005–2010. *BMJ Glob Health*. 2018;3:e000674.
2. Drobac PC, Basinga P, Condo J, et al. Comprehensive and integrated district health systems strengthening: The Rwanda Population Health Implementation and Training (PHIT) Partnership. *BMC Health Serv Res*. 2013;13 Suppl 2(Suppl 2):S5. doi:10.1186/1472-6963-13-S2-S5.
3. World Health Organization. *Everybody's Business: Strengthening Health Systems to Improve Health Outcomes*. Geneva; 2007.
4. Semrau KEA, Hirschhorn LR, Delaney MM, et al. Outcomes of a coaching-based WHO safe childbirth checklist program in India. *N Engl J Med*. 2017;377(24):2313–2324.
5. Conlon CM, Serbanescu F, Marum L, et al. Saving mothers, giving life: It takes a system to save a mother. *Glob Health Sci Pract*. 2019;7(Suppl 1):S6–S26. Published 2019 Mar 13. doi:10.9745/GHSP-D-18-00427.

2

Can Informal Providers Be Trained to Provide Good Quality Care?

SHEGUFTA SHEFA SIKDER

[T]he difficulty of improving the quality of public health care, combined with the scarcity and cost of such doctors, suggests that investing in the clinical practice of informal providers is at least an equally efficient allocation of resources.[1]

Research Question: What is the impact on clinical skills of a multi-topic training program for informal providers?

Funding: Grants from the West Bengal National Rural Health Mission, The World Bank's Knowledge for Change Program, and Bristol-Myers Squibb Foundation Award under the Delivering Hope program to the Liver Foundation, West Bengal, India

Year Study Began: 2012

Year Study Published: 2016

Study Location: Birbhum District in West Bengal, India

Who Was Studied: Informal health providers, identified from a census, who had been practicing allopathic/modern medicine for at least 3 years.

Who Was Excluded: Informal providers who were not living in the villages in which they were working or those who refused to participate.

How Many Subjects: 304 informal providers

Study Overview: See Figure 2.1.

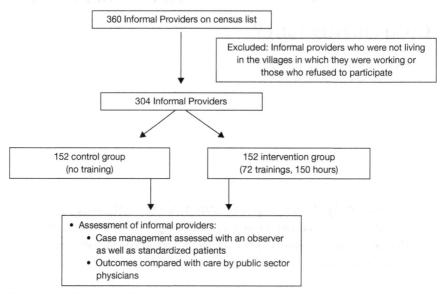

Figure 2.1. Overview of the study design.

Study Intervention: The 304 providers were randomized to a control group and an intervention group (Figure 2.1). The intervention group received training consisting of 72 sessions and 150 teaching hours over a 9-month period. The program offered a generalized curriculum, training providers on multiple topics such as basic physiology and anatomy, harm reduction, and specific illnesses.

After training, visits by unannounced standardized patients and data from day-long clinical observations were used to assess practice. The control group was compared to the intervention group as well as with public-sector physicians practicing in the same village. Three tracer conditions were chosen—chest pain, respiratory distress, and child diarrhea—as proxies for the ability of the informal provider to triage; treat or refer; and assess and treat.

Follow-Up: 9–10 months

Endpoints: Prescription of unnecessary medications or antibiotics, correct management of standardized conditions

RESULTS

- Mean attendance at each training session was 56%.
- Trained providers correctly managed cases 14.2% more than untrained providers. Additionally, the training program reduced the gap in correct case management between informal providers who attended just over half the sessions and physicians in public clinics by half and reduced the gap almost entirely for providers who completed the full course.
- The training had no effect on the use of unnecessary medicines and antibiotics, although both training- and control-group informal providers prescribed 28.2% *fewer* unnecessary antibiotics than public-sector providers.
- The program cost $175 per trainee.
- For trained informal providers, the demand for informal care provider services increased from 15.5% to 28.9% and patient caseload increased by 17%.

Criticisms and Limitations: Providers completed just 52% of sessions. While the authors suppose that coverage could be improved by offering training in more geographically proximate locations, literature suggests that competing time demands often preclude complete involvement of health providers in training. Thus, it is unlikely that results in real-world practice would be better than those demonstrated in this analysis.

Additionally, correct case management was assessed based on three tracer conditions (asthma, diarrhea in children, and chest pain), but the study was not powered to assess correct management of those specific cases. Management of these conditions was extrapolated to indicate general correct case management of typical conditions. While this extrapolation is logical, suppositions and estimates should be interpreted with caution.

Other Relevant Studies and Information:

- Other research in South Asia suggests that competing time demands and high patient load make complete provider participation in trainings challenging.[2,3] While geographic access remains a key consideration, it is not the sole consideration for providers planning their nonclinical time.[4]
- The authors argue that training informal providers may be a worthy investment given that the mean consultation length by public-sector

providers in the public clinic was only 1.74 min. Analyses show that the patient-to-population ratio in India, particularly in states such as Bihar, represent some of the lowest proportions in South Asia,[2] and extrapolating these findings to other locations may not be appropriate.

• There is concern that training of informal providers or "self-proclaimed physicians" despite no formal degree may legitimize these providers and result in worse health outcomes. However, this begs the question of whether training informal providers—even modest training such as the 150 hours in this study—makes them no longer "informal" providers but nonphysician clinicians with a limited scope of practice.

Summary and Implications: In rural settings of South Asia where the availability of formal medical providers may be scant, informal providers commonly provide professional medical services. In this demonstration, a training program for informal providers led to improved case management rates vs. informal providers who did not receive the training. The training was not associated with reduced use of unnecessary medicines or antibiotics, however. Multi-topic medical training for informal providers may offer an effective strategy to improve healthcare access and complement critical investments in the quality of public care.

CLINICAL CASE: IMPROVING ACCESS TO CARE BY TRAINING INFORMAL PROVIDERS

Case History
You are a Ministry of Health employee in a country where the physician-to-patient ratio is 0.003 (the WHO recommends 1 physician per 1000 population). You are tasked with finding creative ways to improve access to care. What are some strategies you could employ based on this chapter and others in this book?

Suggested Answer
With a limited supply of physicians for the population in your country, training and utilization of nonphysician clinicians and informal providers may be a good strategy. Training laypeople from communities to be able to safely triage the most common medical problems within their communities can help divert those who need more care to the few physicians who are available. Utilizing

community members in this way would increase access to culturally competent healthcare within a community and decrease the need for travel and waste of resources for some patients. Additionally, task-shifting of commonly performed procedures, surgeries, or diagnoses to nonphysician clinicians may further improve access to potentially lifesaving interventions. An example would be placing community health workers in villages (training community members to triage, evaluate, and treat or refer for a limited number of issues), and placing nonphysician clinicians who have been trained to offer higher levels of care through task-shifting at local clinics or hospitals, while placing physicians at regional referral centers.

References

1. Das J, Chowdhury A, Hussam R, Banerjee AV. The impact of training informal health care providers in India: A randomized controlled trial. *Science.* 2016;354(6308):aaf7384. doi:10.1126/science.aaf7384. PMID: 27846471.
2. Dieleman M, Gerretsen B, van der Wilt GJ. Human resource management interventions to improve health workers' performance in low and middle income countries: A realist review. *Health Res Policy Sys.* 2009;7:7. doi:10.1186/1478-4505-7-7. PMID: 19374734; PMCID: PMC2672945.
3. Rao M, Rao K, Kumar AS, Chatterjee M, Sundararaman T. Human resources for health in India. *Lancet.* 2011;377(9765):587–598. https://doi.org/10.1016/S0140-6736(10)61888-0.
4. Sikder S, Labrique AB, Ali H, et al. Availability of emergency obstetric care (EmOC) among public and private health facilities in rural northwest Bangladesh. *BMC Public Health.* 2015;15:36. doi:10.1186/s12889-015-1405-2. PMID: 25637319; PMCID: PMC4316389.

3

Can Under-5 Mortality Be Reduced
by Proactive Community Case Management?

*The Effect of Proactive Community Case Management by
Community Health Workers in a Peri-Urban Area in Mali*

VIDIYA SATHANANTHAN AND AMI WATERS

Seven years following the launch of proactive community case management (pro-CCM) [by community health workers (CHWs)] in a peri-urban area, the areas of the intervention had an under-five mortality rate of 7/1000 [down from 154/1000].[1]

Research Question: Does proactive community case management (pro-CCM) of childhood illnesses by community health workers (CHWs) lead to an increase in access to care and reduction in child mortality in a peri-urban setting?

Funding: Child Relief International Foundation

Year Study Began: 2008

Year Study Published: 2018

Study Location: The study was conducted in an approximately 3.5-square-mile peri-urban area of Yirimadio, Mali, outside Bamako.

Who Was Studied: Children 0–59 months visited by CHWs as part of proactive community case management (pro-CCM)

Who Was Excluded: Children over 59 months of age

How Many Patients: 618,877 proactive case finding home visits; 29,561 home visits for sick children 0–59 months old

Study Overview: See Figure 3.1.

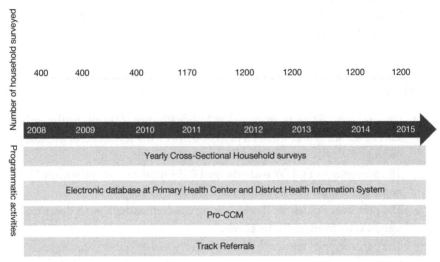

Figure 3.1. Overview of the study design.

Study Intervention: In the treatment group, CHWs conducted proactive community case management (pro-CCM) by searching door-to-door for patients daily. CHWs were trained to diagnose and treat uncomplicated cases of malaria, pneumonia, and diarrhea for children 0–59 months and to refer patients with specified danger signs to the primary health center. CHWs conducted follow-up visits for sick patients at 24, 48, and 72 hours to support adherence and monitor response to therapy. An additional follow-up visit after 5 days was conducted for patients with diarrheal disease. CHWs also performed active case detection and referral of sick newborns, pregnant women, and postpartum women. No user fees were charged for community-based care. CHWs received monthly individual supervision and weekly group supervision. This was also coupled with the improvement of primary care centers. There was no control group in this study.

Follow-Up: 7 years

Endpoints:
Primary outcome:
• Under-5 mortality rate

Secondary outcomes:
- Prevalence of febrile illness among children 0–59 months within the last 2 weeks
- Percentage of febrile children who received effective antimalarial treatment within 24 hours of symptom onset
- Percentage of patients who had a danger or referral sign requiring treatment at the primary care facility[2]
- Percentage of CHW patients aged 0–59 months reached within 24 hours of symptom onset.[3]

RESULTS

- Under-5 mortality was estimated at 154 deaths per 1000 live births at the start of the study and 7 deaths per 1000 live births at the end of the study period.
- The percentage of CHW patients aged 0–59 months reached within 24 hours of symptom onset increased from 25% to 62%.[4,5]
- The prevalence of febrile illness among children under 5 years decreased significantly from 39.7% to 22.6%.
- The percentage of febrile children who received effective antimalarial treatment within 24 hours of symptom onset more than doubled, from 14.7% to 35.3%.

Criticisms and Limitations:

- The study design had no control group and therefore it is not possible to infer causality from this analysis. The observed public health improvements during the study period may have resulted from other concurrent public health interventions.
- The first 2 years of the study were not implemented with sample sizes large enough to appropriately detect under-5 mortality rate. Therefore, the baseline under-5 mortality rate (2008) in this study is likely an overestimate of the true under-5 mortality rate, which may have led to an overestimation of the benefits of the intervention.
- Facility-based interventions, including infrastructure expansion and staff training, were also done as a part of the intervention; thus it is

not possible to determine which components of the intervention were most responsible for the observed benefits.

Other Relevant Studies and Information:

- In 2019 Whidden et al.[2] conducted a systematic review of proactive case detection of common childhood illnesses by CHWs. This analysis found that proactive case detection may reduce infant mortality (RR: 0.52–0.94) compared with conventional healthcare delivery models.
- A 2020 case study of community case management of malaria in Senegal found that introduction of proactive case detection significantly increased detection and treatment of symptomatic malaria cases by CHWs. However, the intervention also highlighted the need to improve the CHW supply chain, supervision, compensation, coordination, and monitoring and evaluation.[3]
- In 2020 Ludwick et al.[4] conducted a systematic review of CHW studies in peri-urban and urban areas, which found that urban CHWs are well-oriented for home visiting and case detection, but more innovation and research are needed to determine the most effective model for utilizing CHWs in urban settings.
- Though numerous studies suggest that integrated community case management may be effective in reducing child mortality, it has been difficult to implement successfully in large-scale national programs, in part due to barriers in the broader system. Community-based interventions including CHWs may be more beneficial in concert with overall health system strengthening efforts.[5]

Summary and Implications: In this analysis in a peri-urban setting in Mali, proactive community case management (pro-CCM) conducted by CHWs, including diagnosis, treatment, and referral for malaria, pneumonia, and diarrhea, was associated with a significant reduction in under-5 mortality rates. This intervention was also associated with increased access to care for children within 24 hours of illness, decreased prevalence of febrile illness among children, and increased receipt of timely, effective antimalarial treatment for children. However, primarily because the study design did not include a control group, it cannot be concluded that the intervention caused these effects; additional rigorous controlled studies are needed. Nevertheless, the findings contribute to current evidence that proactive community case management may be able to reduce under-five mortality and improve child health outcomes in peri-urban settings.

CLINICAL CASE: FOUR-YEAR-OLD FEMALE WITH FEVER IDENTIFIED BY COMMUNITY HEALTH WORKER

Case History

A CHW, Rachel, is doing household visits and comes across a 4-year-old girl who, as reported by the mother, felt hot last night before bed and is now having hot skin this morning. With more questions, the CHW learns that the child is eating well and without vomiting or diarrhea; she has no cough. The patient has not had any convulsions.

Questions

- What illnesses should the CHW be screening for in the community as a part of pro-CCM?
- Should this patient be treated in the community or referred to a clinic?
- When should the CHW follow up with the patient?
- What are some danger signs of malaria for which the CHW should counsel the caregiver that would necessitate going to the facility right away?
- What counseling should the family receive about prevention of malaria?

Suggested Answers

- The patient should be screened for diarrhea, pneumonia, and malaria. Screening for malaria should be with a malaria rapid diagnostic test if available.
- The patient can be treated in the community since she is eating well and thus able to take medicine by mouth.
- The CHW should conduct follow-up visits at 24, 48, and 72 hours since there is no diarrhea.
- If the child is vomiting, unable to keep down medicine, has seizures, or is not able to easily awaken, then the patient should be taken to the clinic right away.
- The family should be reminded to have the child sleep under a bed net, to avoid being outside at dusk, and to keep the area around the home and in the community free of standing water and high grass.

References

1. Johnson AD, Thiero O, Whidden C, et al. Proactive community case management and child survival in periurban Mali. *BMJ Glob Health.* 2018;3:e000634. doi:10.1136/bmjgh-2017-000634

2. Whidden C, Thwing J, Gutman J, et al. Proactive case detection of common childhood illnesses by community health workers: A systematic review. *BMJ Glob Health.* 2019;4(6). doi: 10.1136/bmjgh-2019-001799

3. Gaye S, Kibler J, Ndiaye JL, et al. Proactive community case management in Senegal 2014-2016: A case study in maximizing the impact of community case management of malaria. *Malar J.* 2020 Apr 25;19(1):166. doi:10.1186/s12936-020-03238-0. PMID: 32334581; PMCID: PMC7183580.

4. Ludwick T, Morgan A, Kane S, Kelaher M, Mcpake B. The distinctive roles of urban community health workers in low- and middle-income countries: A scoping review of the literature. *Health Policy Plan.* 2020;35(8):1039–1052. doi:10.1093/heapol/czaa049

5. Daelmans B, Seck A, Nsona H, Wilson S, Young M. Integrated community case management of childhood illness: What have we learned? *Am J Trop Med.* 2016;94(3):571–573. doi: 10.4269/ajtmh.94-3intro2

4

A Participatory Intervention with Women's Groups for Reducing Neonatal Mortality and Maternal Depression

The Ekjut Trial

SHYAMSUNDAR J. RAITHATHA

Women's groups led by peer facilitators reduced NMR [neonatal mortality rate] and moderate maternal depression at low cost in [a] largely tribal, rural population of eastern India.
—EKJUT TRIAL INVESTIGATOR TEAM[1]

Research Question: Can a participatory intervention with women's groups in underserved tribal communities of eastern India improve neonatal and peripartum health outcomes?

Funding: Health Foundation, UK; Department for International Development, Wellcome Trust; and Big Lottery Fund, UK

Year Study Began: 2005

Year Study Published: 2010

Study Location: 3 tribal districts of 2 of the poorest states (Jharkhand and Orissa) of eastern India

Who Was Studied: Women age 15–49 years who had given birth during the study period.

Who Was Excluded: Women who refused interviews and women who migrated out from the study population.

How Many Participants: 17,035 mothers (see details in Table 4.1)

Table 4.1 Number of Participants for Outcomes Measurement
and the Intervention

Participant	Intervention	Control
For outcomes measurement		
Clusters (mean cluster population: 6338)	18	18
Mothers	8743	8292
Births	9770	9260
For intervention		
Women's groups	241	NA
Group attendances over 3 years	111 006	
Married women in reproductive age group in group attendances	74 715 (67%)	
Adolescent girls in group attendances	15 030 (14%)	
Elderly women in group attendances	10 809 (10%)	

Study Overview: See Figure 4.1.

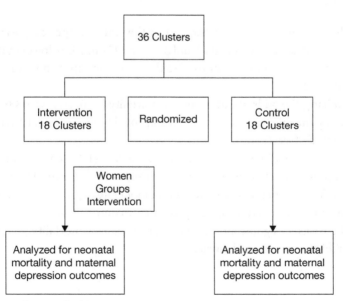

Figure 4.1. Ekjut study design.

Study Intervention: In the 18 intervention clusters, 244 women's groups (172 preexisting and 72 newly created) were the focus of intervention using a participatory learning and action cycle (PLA). There was an average of one group per 468 population. Anyone from the population could attend the meetings. Each group met monthly for 20 meetings facilitated by a local woman identified as a facilitator. Information about clean delivery practices and care–seeking behavior was shared using case studies through stories, picture–card games, and role–play. Based on this information, group members prioritized maternal and neonatal health problems and identified and implemented relevant strategies to address them. Each group was free to implement its own combination of strategies with a few common approaches.

These results were adjusted for stratification, clustering, maternal education, assets, and any tribal affiliation.

In the control clusters, there was no facilitation of women's groups.

Follow-Up: 3 years

Endpoints:

Primary endpoints: Neonatal mortality and maternal depression

Secondary endpoints: Stillbirth, perinatal death, maternal death, uptake of antenatal and delivery services, home-care practices (during and after deliveries), and health-seeking behavior.

RESULTS

- The odds of neonatal mortality during the year study period (years 1–3) and last 2 years (years 2 and 3) were 32% and 45% lower in the intervention group as compared to the control group, respectively (see Table 4.2).
- Similarly, the odds of early neonatal mortality (0–6 days) was 38% lower during the full 3-year study period and 54% lower in the final 2 years of the study (see Table 4.2).
- There was no difference in maternal depression (K10 score) during the study period between the intervention and control groups. However, in year 3, a 57% reduction in the odds of moderate depression was noted in the intervention group as compared to the control group.
- There was no significant reduction in late neonatal mortality (7–28 days), stillbirths, or maternal mortality.

Table 4.2 SUMMARY OF FINDINGS

Variable	Adjusted OR (95% CI) Years 1–3	Adjusted OR (95% CI) Years 2 and 3	Adjusted OR (95% CI) Year 2	Adjusted OR (95% CI) Year 3
Neonatal mortality	0.68 (0.59–0.78)	0.55 (0.46–0.66)	NA	NA
Early neonatal mortality (0–6 days)	0.62 (0.52–0.73)	0.46 (0.37–0.57)	NA	NA
Late neonatal mortality (7–28 days)	0.84 (0.64–1.12)	0.80 (0.56–1.14)	NA	NA
Stillbirth	1.05 (0.86–1.28)	1.01 (0.80–1.28)	NA	NA
Perinatal mortality	0.79 (0.69–0.91)	0.68 (0.58–0.79)	NA	NA
Maternal mortality	0.70 (0.46–1.07)	0.50 (0.48–1.49)	NA	NA
No or mild depression	NA	1.29 (0.68–2.44)	0.91 (0.41–2.01)	2.33 (1.25–4.38)
Moderate depression	NA	0.74 (0.40–1.37)	1.04 (0.50–2.16)	0.43 (0.23–0.80)
Severe depression	NA	1.29 (0.46–3.64)	1.53 (0.47–5.05)	0.70 (0.15–3.31)

Criticisms and Limitations:

- Although neonatal mortality improved as a result of the intervention, there was no observed improvement in home care practices, raising questions about the mechanism of these mortality improvements.
- This study was conducted during a time period when home deliveries were common in eastern India; since this time, institutional deliveries have become more common, raising questions about the continued applicability of these study results.

Other Relevant Studies and Information:

- In a cluster-randomized controlled trial performed in a poor, rural population in Nepal,[2] the authors show a 30% reduction in the odds of neonatal mortality utilizing PLA. In addition, they saw an improvement in health-service utilization for antenatal care and institutional deliveries.

- A meta-analysis of cluster-randomized trials[3] was performed to analyze the ways that PLA may lead to a reduction in neonatal mortality. The researchers found a correlation between improvements in health outcomes and better home-care behaviors, including an increase in the use of safe delivery kits and use of a sterile blade to cut the umbilical cord; birth attendant washing hands prior to delivery; delayed bathing of the newborn for at least 24 hours; and wrapping the newborn within 10 minutes of delivery.
- The World Health Organization (WHO) recommends that the community be mobilized through the utilization of PLA with women's groups to improve maternal and newborn health, particularly in rural settings with low access to health services.[4]

Summary and Implications: This trial found that a community intervention, PLA, involving women's groups for new mothers in rural communities in eastern India, was associated with a significant reduction (32%) in the odds of neonatal mortality. The PLA is a proven method and can be adapted for behavior change for other health problems. As the proportion of institutional deliveries increases, different approaches for improving neonatal mortality shall have to be explored.

CLINICAL CASE: HEALTH SYSTEMS STRENGTHENING

Case History

You are working on a health systems improvement project in collaboration with the government, focusing on improving neonatal mortality in a deprived tribal district. The neonatal mortality rates and percentage of home deliveries are among the highest in the country. The indigenous population prefers delivery by traditional birth attendants (TBA) who have no formal training in infection control or evidence-based management of deliveries. The government doesn't accept the TBAs and has been incentivizing its community health workers (CHWs) to improve institutional deliveries to no avail. Based on the above study, how might you mobilize the community to improve neonatal mortality, and what issues might you encounter?

Suggested Answer

The WHO recommends utilizing a PLA intervention with women's groups to improve neonatal mortality. For any community intervention, political support is essential, and the intervention must be adapted to reflect the locale's

context, capacity, and constraints. For example, implementation should consider the role of men and other members of the community such as religious
groups or elders and mothers-in-law, and how and when they should participate in the process, as well as preferences for oral vs. visual methods, level of
literacy, etc. You would need to build relationships with local tribal leaders,
traditional birth attendants, and other stakeholders to create a space for discussion where women are able to identify priority problems and advocate for local
solutions for maternal and newborn health.

In this particular case, empowering pregnant women, key community
members, and TBAs with knowledge and training on evidence-based birth
practices, as well as working with them to develop referral protocols during
delivery, may help reduce neonatal mortality, as discussed in the study and
further reading above. To have an impact, the time period of the intervention should be no shorter than 3 years (which was the follow-up period
in this study). Of note, cooperation from non-health sectors may be crucial for implementing group plans (e.g., road development to aid in timely
transfer).

References

1. Tripathy P, Nair N, Barnett S, et al. Effect of a participatory intervention with women's
   groups on birth outcomes and maternal depression in Jharkhand and Orissa, India: A
   cluster-randomised controlled trial. *Lancet*. 2010;375(9721):1182–1192.
2. Manandhar DS, Osrin D, Shrestha BP, et al. Effect of a participatory intervention with
   women's groups on birth outcomes in Nepal: Cluster-randomised controlled trial.
   Lancet. 2004;364(9438):970–979.
3. Seward N, Neuman M, Colbourn T, et al. Effects of women's groups practising participatory learning and action on preventive and care-seeking behaviours to reduce neonatal mortality: A meta-analysis of cluster-randomised trials. *PLoS Med*.
   2017;14(12):e1002467.
4. World Health Organization. WHO recommendation on community mobilization
   through facilitated participatory learning and action cycles with women's groups for
   maternal and newborn health. World Health Organization; 2014. https://apps.who.
   int/iris/handle/10665/127939

5

A Case Management Strategy for Treating Childhood Pneumonia in a Community Setting?

JENNIFER WERDENBERG

The consistency of findings across all the studies . . . shows that case-management strategy has a substantial effect on infant and under-5 mortality, at least in settings with infant mortality rates of 90/1000 live births or more.[1]

Research Question: Is the pneumonia case-management strategy proposed by World Health Organization (WHO), which relies on community health workers' ability to recognize, diagnose, and presumptively treat pneumonia, effective at improving child survival?

Funding: WHO Acute Respiratory Infections Control Program, USAID, Rockefeller Foundation

Year Study Began: Included studies began 1985–1987

Year Study Published: 1992

Study Location: Studies included were conducted in Bangladesh, Pakistan, India, Nepal, and Tanzania

Who Was Studied: Intervention studies which used the WHO case management approach for pneumonia in children under 5 years of age were included.

Who Was Excluded: Intervention studies outside this age-group or studies employing strategies other than the WHO case management approach were excluded.

How Many Patients Studied: Total child years studied:
- 0–1 year: 48 695
- 1–4 years: 160 933

Study Overview: Figure 5.1 summarizes the study design. The included studies were either community-based randomized controlled trials or pre-post studies.

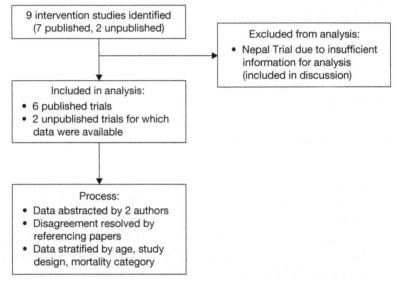

Figure 5.1. Overview of the study design.

Study Intervention: Description of meta-analysis strategy:

- Cochrane method as modified by Desimonian and Laird was used for estimation of confidence limits for the risk differences in individual studies and for summary estimates of impact across studies.
  Method produces weighted average of the rate differences (weight determined by inverse combination of variation within and between studies)
- Homogeneity of intervention effect across studies assessed with Cochrane's Q test.
- If substantial heterogeneity among stratum specific estimates was seen, the results were confirmed by the Miettinen method.
- Homogeneity evaluated by the Breslow and Day method.

Description of interventions included in data for meta-analysis: The interventions included utilizing the WHO case management of pneumonia approach for children under 5, which involves empiric antibiotic treatment for *S. pneumonia* and *H. influenzae* pneumonia based on an algorithmic diagnosis of pneumonia in children with cough, high respiratory rate, and chest in-drawing as recognized by health workers.

In addition to pneumonia, some of the included studies also had co-management of other conditions, such as:

- Diarrhea with oral rehydration solutions (ORS)
- Education on family planning and maternal health
- Immunization
- Vitamin A supplementation
- Referral of severely sick children
- Nutritional rehabilitation.

Follow-Up: Up to 4 years

RESULTS

- Rate difference
  - Infant mortality overall rate reduction was 15.9% (95% CI 10.6–21.1) deaths/1000 live births
  - Mortality rate in children under-5 decreased by 36 deaths/1000 live births.
  - Pooled estimate infant mortality due to lower respiratory infections was reduced by 10.7 (4.8–16.7) deaths/1000 live births
- Pooled estimates of relative risk
  - 20% reduction in infant mortality
  - 25% reduction in under-5 mortality.

Criticisms and Limitations:

- Studies examined and included reported child deaths from acute lower respiratory infection (ALRI), which is presumed to be primarily due to pneumonia; however, the range of etiologies for ALRI in infants under 5 years of age is broad, especially when not excluding the neonatal period as in some studies.
- While community case management continues to be an important underpinning of the global strategy to mitigate under-5 death, the effect

of this isolated intervention, which was concluded to be significant in settings with infant mortality rates of 90/1000 live births or more, should be applied thoughtfully to appropriate populations.

Other Relevant Studies and Information:

- This meta-analysis is cited as foundational in the development of the integrated management of childhood illness (IMCI) in 1995, which targeted (what were at the time) the 5 most important causes of child mortality: acute respiratory infection, diarrhea, measles, malaria, and malnutrition.[2]
- In 2013 Das et al.[3] conducted a systematic review of all randomized controlled trials, quasi-experimental, and observational studies to estimate the effect of community-based interventions on mortality due to pneumonia and diarrhea. Results showed a 32% decrease in pneumonia-specific mortality secondary to these interventions.

Summary and Implications: This meta-analysis demonstrated that a case management strategy for evaluating and treating children with pneumonia in a community setting can effectively lower childhood mortality, particularly in low-resource settings with high baseline child mortality rates.

CLINICAL CASE: COMMUNITY HEALTH WORKER (CHW) UTILIZES INTEGRATED MANAGEMENT OF CHILDHOOD ILLNESS STRATEGY TO ASSESS A SICK CHILD AT HOME

Case History

Grace, a community health worker in a rural village in Rwanda, does her monthly check-in on children under the age of 5 years.

Shining is a 17-month-old girl whose mother is concerned she is not eating enough. Shining is breastfeeding without chest in-drawing when Grace walks in; she has yellow-green discharge from her nose and a wet cough. Her mom does not think she felt warm, has not had any seizures, diarrhea, or rashes, and has needed her nappy changed at least 4 times yesterday. She has had nasal discharge and decreased appetite for about 2 days. Shining's respiratory rate is 50 breaths per minute, and she walks unsteadily around the house, breathing slightly heavily but without stridor, while Grace completes education with the mother.

- What elements of IMCI has the child screened positively for?
- Should the case worker refer or manage at home?
- What interventions that the community health worker can provide should be started now regardless of the decision to refer or not?

Suggested Answer

IMCI addresses acute respiratory infection, diarrhea, measles, malaria, and malnutrition. Steps for CHWs to utilize IMCI tools are: (1) assess; (2) classify need for urgent referral, specific medical treatment, or home management; (3) identify treatment; (4) treat; (5) counsel; and (6) follow up.

- Assess: For danger signs (inability to drink/breastfeeding, vomiting everything, convulsions, lethargy, unconscious) indicative of a life-threatening condition
- Classify: Grace performed a focused physical exam in which she determined that the child was well nourished and able to breastfeed but did have signs of non-severe pneumonia.
- Identify treatment: Treatment of non-severe pneumonia in Grace's district is co-trimoxazole for 5 days.
- Treat: She administers the first dose of the drug to the child while teaching the mother how to give future doses. Additionally, she encourages the mother to breastfeed.
- Counsel: Grace educates Shining's mother on danger signs, how to watch for chest in-drawing.
- Follow-up: Grace educates Shining's mother on the location of the nearest clinic in case Shining worsens over the next 1–2 days.

References

1. Sazawal S, Black R. Meta-analysis of intervention trials on case-management of pneumonia in community settings. *Lancet*. 1992;340:528–533.
2. Campbell H, Gove S. Integrated management of childhood infections and malnutrition: A global initiative. *Arch Dis Child*. 1996;75:468–471.
3. Das JK, Lassi ZS, Salam RA, Bhutta ZA. Effect of community based interventions on childhood diarrhea and pneumonia: Uptake of treatment modalities and impact on mortality. *BMC Public Health*. 2013;13(Suppl 3):S29.

6

Can Checklists Improve Perinatal Outcomes?

The Better Birth Trial

ANDREA WALKER

[W]e found that the BetterBirth program—a coaching-based implementation of the WHO Safe Child-birth Checklist—had no significant effect on . . . maternal and perinatal health (nor on any secondary
health outcomes), despite significantly higher rates of birth attendants'
adherence to essential practices in intervention facilities than in control
facilities.

—SEMRAU ET AL.[1]

Research Question: Can implementation of an evidence-based birthing practices
checklist improve perinatal mortality and morbidity in under-resourced areas?

Funding: Bill and Melinda Gates Foundation, Clinical Trials number
NCT02148952

Year Study Began: November 2014

Year Study Published: December 2017

Study Location: Uttar Pradesh, India

Who Was Studied: Women delivering at government-run primary health
centers, community health centers, or first referral facilities.

Who Was Excluded: Women who delivered outside of the hospital, women referred from other facilities, and those undergoing abortion. Also excluded were women delivering at government facilities with lower volume or few providers with requisite midwifery training, or facilities that were already unable or unwilling to fully engage in the study.

How Many Participants: 120 facilities were included with a total of 157 689 eligible patients

Study Overview: Figure 6.1 provides an overview of the study design.

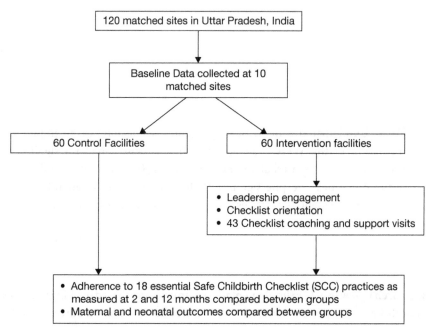

Figure 6.1. Overview of the study design.

Study intervention: Intervention facilities received paper copies of the Safe Childbirth Checklist (SCC). Although the SCC includes 28 best practices, for the purposes of the study, adherence to 18 essential practices was studied, as shown in Box 6.1. To facilitate use of the checklist, the intervention facilities received coaching in understanding and implementing the checklist: nursing coaches conducted 43 visits to each intervention facility over an 8-month time frame. Physician or public health professional Coach Team Leaders also attended half of these visits. A childbirth quality coordinator was chosen from each site to perform continued on-site coaching and troubleshoot any barriers to checklist implementation. The control facilities provided their current standard of care but were similarly monitored for their adherence to the 18 essential practices as outlined in the SCC.

BOX 6.1 THE 18 ESSENTIAL BIRTH PRACTICES MONITORED IN THIS STUDY

Before birth:
- Birth companion present*
- Partography started

Before pushing:
- Hand hygiene
- Clean towel available
- Clean scissors or blade available*
- Cord tie available*
- Mucus extractor available*
- Neonatal bag and mask available*
- Pads available

Within 1 minute after delivery:
- Oxytocin administered
- Birth companion present*

Within 1 hour after delivery:
- Newborn weight taken*
- Newborn temperature taken*
- Skin-to-skin care initiated at birth
- Skin-to-skin care maintained for 1 hour
- Initiation of breastfeeding

*There was no significant difference in adherence to these practices between the control or intervention sites at 2 or 12 months.

Follow-Up: 7 days postpartum

Endpoints:

Primary outcome: A composite measure of perinatal death, maternal death, or maternal severe complications (including seizures, loss of consciousness >1 hour, fever with foul-smelling vaginal discharge, hemorrhage or stroke) within 7 days of delivery.

Secondary outcomes: Maternal secondary outcomes included maternal death, referral, cesarean section, hysterectomy, blood transfusion, and readmission within 7 days after delivery. Neonatal secondary outcomes included stillbirth, early neonatal death, and interfacility transfer.

RESULTS

- At 2 months into the study, overall adherence to the 18 essential practices was significantly higher in the intervention group compared to the control group (72.8% vs. 41.7%) (Table 6.1).
- At 12 months into the study (4 months after coaching ended), checklist adherence to the 18 essential practices dropped to 61.7% vs. 43.9% at the intervention and control sites, respectively (Table 6.1).
- Adherence to some individual practices remained at statistically significantly higher levels in the intervention sites than the control sites at 12 months, including: starting partography on admission, administration of oxytocin, hand hygiene, initiation and maintenance of skin-to-skin, breastfeeding, and administration of postpartum maternal vitals (Table 6.1).
- Despite an increase in checklist adherence in the intervention sites, there were not any significant improvements in perinatal or maternal outcomes.

Table 6.1 SUMMARY OF KEY FINDINGS

Checklist Adherence	% Adherence Intervention	Control	P value
2 months	72.8	41.7	<0.001
12 months	61.7	43.9	<0.001
Clinical Outcomes	**Relative Risk for Intervention Group Compared with Control Group** (95% CI)		
Primary Outcome (*composite* measure of perinatal death, maternal death, or maternal severe complications)	0.99 (0.83–1.18)		
Secondary Outcome (severe maternal complications or severe neonatal complications)	1.03 (0.89–1.20)		

Criticisms and Limitations:

- The effort to accurately capture SCC adherence was limited by Hawthorne effect, the number of births witnessed (2% of the total), and lack of any night shift data.

- The adherence outcome does not take into account the differential impact of the checklist items. Having a birth companion present may be less impactful on outcomes than measuring blood pressure.
- The Better Birth Trial encouraged the utilization of these 18 "best practices" which would serve to fill knowledge gaps on the part of providers and act as reminders in providing care. However, the program did not address gaps that occur as a result of lack of resources (medications, equipment, infrastructure).

Other Relevant Studies:

- The checklist strategy has now permeated other areas of healthcare delivery with some success.[2–5] For example, the WHO Safe Surgery Checklist has been shown to consistently reduce perioperative mortality. Implementation of a "sign in," "time out," and "sign out" reduced the death rate from 1.5% to 0.8% (p = 0.003).[5] In contrast to the Better Birth study above, the Safe Surgery study heavily relied on local staff and a multidisciplinary team approach incorporating nurses, surgeons, anesthetists, and patients.
- Taking a different approach from that seen in the Better Birth study, Youngelson et al. partnered with and strengthened a health system in South Africa by focusing on multiple levels of healthcare: boosting multidisciplinary quality improvement initiatives, changing policies and protocols across all levels of pregnancy care, and focusing on acquisition and maintenance of necessary supplies and equipment. With this broad approach, they successfully reduced mother-to-child HIV transmission from 7.6% to 5%.[6]
- Despite a reported global increase in facility-based births, maternal and neonatal mortality rates have not improved in low- and middle-income countries (LMICs). Strategies to target this metric for further improvement have remained challenging given the vast array of contributors to obstetric outcomes. It is likely that any improvement in mortality or morbidity will require a complex set of interventions on multiple levels.[7,8]

Summary and Implications: Despite implementation of an obstetrical safety checklist in birthing facilities in under-resourced regions of India and resulting improvements in adherence to evidence-based safety practices in the peripartum period, there was no improvement in maternal or neonatal outcomes. These results suggest that the use of an obstetrical checklist in isolation may not be sufficient to improve birthing outcomes.

CLINICAL CASE: UNDERSTANDING THE COMPLEXITY OF HEALTH SYSTEMS AND APPLYING A SYSTEMS-LEVEL ANALYSIS WHEN DESIGNING INTERVENTIONS

Case History

You are a consultant with an NGO in rural India. The region you are in has high levels of maternal death. You are tasked with designing an intervention to decrease the maternal death rate. What factors would you consider in designing your interventions?

Suggested Answer

As discussed above, best practice checklists have been shown to improve outcomes before; however, it is also clear that maternal and neonatal morbidity and mortality are governed by complex processes and may require interventions at all levels of a health system. A strategic framework has been proposed that works to integrate services in a way that increases efficiency and value for the patient, while reducing overall healthcare costs. It details four levels of intervention,[8] including:

1. Integrating care with other independent conditions
2. Using shared delivery infrastructure across multiple medical conditions to maximize cooperation and collaboration between personnel and facilities when working to prevent and treat conditions
3. Incorporating local knowledge
4. Designing healthcare delivery systems to maximize their contribution to equitable economic and community development.

Additionally, the "4 S's" have been proposed as vital components of global health development: stuff (medical equipment), staff (properly trained and compensated healthcare professionals), space (clean and sanitary patient care environment), and systems (infrastructure).8 Addressing these 4 S's and thereby attending to multiple levels of a health system could help tackle this complex issue. Together, these frameworks could be considered and employed in this setting to strengthen the health system comprehensively and improve outcomes.

References

1. Semrau KEA, Hirschhorn LR, Kodkany B, et al. Effectiveness of the WHO Safe Childbirth Checklist program in reducing severe maternal, fetal, and newborn harm in Uttar Pradesh, India: Study protocol for a matched-pair, cluster-randomized controlled trial. *Trials.* 2016;17:576.

2. Gawande A. *Checklist Manifesto: How to Get Things Right*. Metropolitan Books; 2009.

3. van Klei WA, Hoff RG, van Aarnhem EE, et al. Effects of the introduction of the WHO "Surgical Safety Checklist" on in-hospital mortality: A cohort study. *Ann Surg.* 2012 Jan;255(1):44–9.

4. Ko HC, Turner TJ, Finnigan MA. Systematic review of safety checklists for use by medical care teams in acute hospital settings: Limited evidence of effectiveness. *BMC Health Serv Res.* 2011 Sep 2;11:211.

5. Haynes AB, Weiser TG, Berry WR, Lipsitz SR, Gawande AA; Safe Surgery Saves Lives Study Group. A surgical safety checklist to reduce morbidity and mortality in a global population. *N Engl J Med.* 2009 Jan 29;360(5):491–499.

6. Youngleson MS, Nkurunziza P, Jennings K, Arendse J, Mate KS, Barker P. Improving a mother to child HIV transmission programme through health system redesign: Quality improvement, protocol adjustment and resource addition. *PLoS One.* 2010 Nov 9;5(11):e13891.

7. Dettrick Z, Firth S, Jimenez Soto E. Do strategies to improve quality of maternal and child health care in lower and middle income countries lead to improved outcomes? A review of the evidence. *PLoS One.* 2013;8(12):e83070.

8. Farmer P. Kellogg Institute for International Studies. Notre Dame; 2016, April. Retrieved from https://science.nd.edu/news/solving-the-ebola-outbreak-paul-farmer-and-the-four-ss/

7

The SimCard Trial

RODRIGO BAZUA LOBATO

The SimCard trial provided clear evidence of the simplified cardiovascular management program's effectiveness in increasing the proportion of high-risk individuals taking antihypertensive medication and aspirin.

—THE SIMCARD INVESTIGATORS[1]

Research Question: Can community health workers (CHWs) increase the proportion of individuals appropriately receiving antihypertensive treatment, as well as a number of secondary outcomes, in resource-scarce regions?

Funding: The US National Heart, Lung, and Blood Institute, National Institutes of Health, Department of Health and Human Services

Year Study Began: 2012

Year Published: 2015

Study Location: 27 rural villages in Tibet and 20 rural villages in Haryana State, India.

Who Was Studied: Residents of the participating villages who had high cardiovascular risk. High cardiovascular risk was defined as individuals age 40 years or older with self-reported history of coronary heart disease (cardiovascular diseases [CVD]), stroke, diabetes, and/or measured systolic blood pressure ≥160 mmHg.

Who Was Excluded: Individuals who had CVD-related complications that could not be managed in a primary care setting, had a malignancy or life-threatening disease, individuals who were bedridden or were participating in any other clinical trial at the same time, and anyone unable to stay in the village longer than 8 months out of the year.

How Many Patients: 2086

Study Overview: See Figure 7.1.

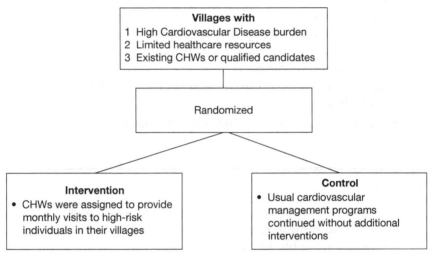

Figure 7.1. Summary of SimCard design.

Study Intervention: Villages were randomized into control (23) and intervention (24) groups. In the control group, the usual cardiovascular management programs continued without additional interventions.

In the intervention group, CHWs were assigned to provide monthly visits to high-risk individuals in their villages. Visits included screening for new symptoms, diseases, and side effects since the last visit, measuring blood pressure, providing lifestyle counseling, and when appropriate, prescribing one or two medications. CHWs were assisted by a mobile-technology-based decision-support system (Electronic Decision Support System [EDSS]) in a smartphone.

CHWs could prescribe two therapeutic lifestyle modifications (smoking cessation and salt reduction) and two medications: a low-dose antihypertensive drug (hydrochlorothiazide 12.5 mg/day in Tibet and a calcium channel blocker 2.5 or 5 mg/day in India) and aspirin 75 mg/day. All hypertensive patients (systolic blood pressure [SBP] >140) without contraindications would be prescribed the antihypertensive medication with a target 140 mmHg or lower. Only patients with coronary heart disease, ischemic stroke, and diabetes, but without contraindications such as bleeding or SBP >160, would be prescribed aspirin.

Follow-Up: 1 year

Endpoints:

Primary outcome: Net difference between groups in the change in the proportion of patient-reported antihypertensive medication use from baseline to 1-year follow-up.

Secondary outcomes:
- The proportion of participants taking aspirin
- Mean systolic blood pressures of participants
- The proportion of current smokers
- The proportion of participants receiving monthly follow-ups from the CHWs
- The proportion of high-risk individuals hospitalized.

RESULTS

- In the intervention group, the proportion of individuals taking antihypertensive medication went from less than 7% to 36.3%. No difference was identified in the control group.
- There was a 17.1% net increase in the proportion of high-risk individuals taking aspirin (24.5% in China and 9.8% in India) in the intervention group.
- A decrease of 2.7 mmHg in mean SBP was identified in the intervention group (4.1 mmHg in Tibet but no change in India).
- Both regions had a >16% net increase in the proportion of high-risk patients receiving monthly follow-up.

Criticism and Limitations: From the perspective of program design, there were several elements of high-quality CHW programs that were lacking in the study. CHWs in the study received only a brief training and very little supervision and were not part of data feedback loops. Even though the EDSS was mentioned as a support tool for CHWs, there is no further description of it in the article. The role of the support app is unclear given that the intervention is very simple and has few decision ramifications from the initial assessment. Due to the weak design of the CHW program in this study, it is possible that stronger CHW programs may offer better clinical results.

Other Relevant Studies and Information:

- CHW programs have been proven effective in improving a variety of clinical outcomes. For example, the use of CHWs has been shown to reduce child mortality in areas with high infant mortality.[2]
- The effectiveness of CHW programs is influenced by the context of implementation, which should be considered in the design of programs.[3] Context includes social and cultural norms, disease-related stigma, safety and security, education and knowledge level of the target group, geography and climate, health service functionality, and local and national politics, among others.
- Existing evidence suggests that, compared with standard care, using CHWs in health programs has the potential to be effective in LMICs, particularly for tobacco cessation and blood pressure and diabetes control.[4,5]

Summary and Implications: In areas with limited primary-care infrastructure and services, such as the rural and marginalized populations analyzed in the study, properly trained CHWs can provide basic treatment at the doorstep of patients, supported by m-health protocols to help them in the decision-making process. The major effect found in the study was an increase of patients with CVD taking evidence-based pharmacologic treatment, but there was no effect on lifestyle modifications.

PUBLIC HEALTH CASE: EXPANDING THE EFFECTIVE COVERAGE OF HEALTHCARE IN REMOTE REGIONS

Case History

Bolivia is analyzing how to provide clinical care in a rural area with a high prevalence of CVD. The majority of the population are low-income farmers. There is very little health infrastructure in the region, and a low ratio of health providers in the region.

Based on the results of the study, how would you expand the effective health coverage of the population in the region?

Suggested Answer

The study demonstrated that CHWs supported by mobile technology can expand the coverage of CVD risk management. Thus, a CHW program could be implemented in the region to rapidly expand health coverage. CHWs could provide basic pharmacologic treatment and identify patients that needed prompt referral. To strengthen the findings of the study, CHWs could be paid and accredited, continuously trained, supported by a dedicated supervisor and part of a data feedback loop. At the same time, the health system should be strengthened so that CHWs could refer patients that they may not be able to treat in their community.

References

1. Tian M, Ajay VS, Dunzhu D, et al. A cluster-randomized, controlled trial of a simplified multifaceted management program for individuals at high cardiovascular risk (SimCard Trial) in Rural Tibet, China, and Haryana, India. *Circulation.* 2015 Sep 1;132(9):815–824. doi:10.1161/CIRCULATIONAHA.115.015373. Epub 2015 Jul 17. PMID: 26187183; PMCID: PMC4558306.
2. Johnson AD, Thiero O, Whidden C, et al. Proactive community case management and child survival in periurban Mali. *BMJ Global Health.* 2018;3(2):e000634.
3. Kok MC, Kane SS, Tulloch O, et al. How does context influence performance of community Health workers in low-and middle-income countries? Evidence from the literature. *Health Res Policy Syst.* 2015;13(1):13.
4. Kim K, Choi JS, Choi E, et al. Effects of community-based health worker interventions to improve chronic disease management and care among vulnerable populations: A systematic review. *Am J Public Health.* 2016 Apr;106(4):e3–e28.
5. Jeet G, Thakur JS, Prinja S, Singh M. Community health workers for non-communicable diseases prevention and control in developing countries: Evidence and implications. *PLoS One.* 2017 Jul 13;12(7):e0180640.

8

DOTS-Plus

Advent of Outpatient Care for MDR-TB

TUSHAR GARG

Community-Based Therapy for Multidrug-Resistant Tuberculosis in Lima, Peru[1]

> Our experience establishes that patients with chronic multidrug-resistant tuberculosis (MDR-TB)[2] can be treated successfully as outpatients outside referral centers and in a resource-poor country.
>
> —MITNICK ET AL.[1]

Research Question: Is community-based, ambulatory treatment feasible for treating multidrug-resistant tuberculosis (MDR-TB) in a low-resource setting?

Funding: Thomas J. White, the Massachusetts State Laboratory Institute; National Institute of Allergy and Infectious Diseases; Eli Lilly; Bill and Melinda Gates Foundation

Year Study Began: 1996

Year Study Published: 2003

Study Location: Lima, Peru

Who Was Studied: TB patients with lab-confirmed MDR-TB who were referred after treatment failed with at least one cycle of directly observed, standardized short-course (DOTS) therapy.

Who Was Excluded: People who died before results of drug-susceptibility testing were available.

How Many Patients: 75

Study Overview: See Figure 8.1.

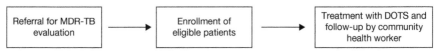

Figure 8.1. Overview of the study design.

Study Intervention: The intervention called DOTS-Plus provides individualized treatment based on drug-susceptibility testing (DST) administered under direct observation in an outpatient setting. It is complemented with monthly sputum cultures and clinical evaluation, treatment, and adverse events monitoring by a trained clinical team that included community health workers (CHWs), and nutritional, financial, and social support.

Follow-Up: 40 months

Endpoints:
 Primary outcome: Number of patients with probable cure, defined as at least 12 consecutive negative monthly sputum cultures during treatment.
 Secondary outcome: Risk factors associated with poor outcome, defined as treatment failure or death.

RESULTS

- Out of the 66 patients completing 4 or more months of treatment, 55 (83%) achieved probable cure; 44 (73%) of the 60 patients whose records were reviewed reported adverse events (Table 8.1).
- Risk factors associated with time to poor outcome included: low hematocrit (adjusted hazard ratio: 4.09, 95% CI: 1.35–12.36), low body mass index (aHR: 3.23, 95% CI: 0.90–11.53), pyrazinamide and ethambutol in regimen of eligible patients (aHR: 0.30, 95% CI: 0.11–0.83) (Table 8.1).

Table 8.1 SUMMARY OF PATIENT OUTCOMES

Patient Outcomes in the Study Indicator	Patients ($n = 75$)
Completed therapy ≥4 months	66
Probable cure	55 (83%)

Criticisms and Limitations:

- This study invested significant resources into the program, which may not be possible in many resource-denied settings. For example, in this study some samples for DST were flown to a high-income country for testing, in-country testing was performed by staff from a high-income country, intensive clinical monitoring was performed, and multiple international academic and nonprofit institutions provided support.
- Although TB programs in low-resource settings are rapidly moving toward outpatient care for drug-resistant TB in the two decades since this study, individualized therapy and person-centered care are still not easily available due to resource constraints.

Other Relevant Studies and Information:

- DST, particularly for patients in whom treatment has failed previously, with DST-guided chemotherapy offered in a community-based, person-centered care setting, can be expected to improve patient outcomes by maximizing the benefits of currently available tools.
- A similar approach improved outcomes in people with extensively drug-resistant (XDR) TB[2] in Peru with 60% ($n = 29/48$) of patients either completing treatment or achieving cure.[3] It also worked for children with MDR-TB where 95% ($n = 36/38$) of the children achieved a favorable outcome.[4]
- In this study cohort, side effects could be managed in an outpatient setting and life-threatening events were rare.[5]
- Besides a strong TB program, program components like comprehensive care in a community-based setting, a well-trained team, and tackling inequity were critical to the success of the DOTS-Plus program.[6]

Summary and Implications: The DOTS-Plus program for people with drug-resistant TB provided individualized, person-centered care in a community-based, outpatient setting in a low-resource environment and was associated with a >80% success rate. This study catalyzed changes to guidelines and practice of treating every drug-resistant case in an in-patient hospital setting.[7,8] It also highlighted the limits of the standardized short-course approach to TB treatment.

PROGRAMMATIC AND POLICY CASE: IMPROVING TB CARE WITHOUT FURTHER BURDENING HOSPITALS

Case History

A low-income country has found an opportunity to improve TB care in its national program through a loan program offered to its government. An infectious disease physician trained in the Global North leads the loan program but has no experience of treating TB in resource-constrained regions. The physician suggests bolstering the hospital-based treatment for drug-resistant TB. How might this study influence that mindset?

Suggested Answer

The case for investment in hospitals catering to people with TB is justified, but only for a subset of cases which are complicated, cannot be ambulatorily managed, or those who require hospitalization after adverse events. The patients within the existing program will benefit more from increasing the DST capacity, strengthening the community-based care for drug-resistant TB, improving patient support systems, and enhancing capacity to report and manage adverse events. The program should consider expanding this model of care to all age groups and forms of TB.

While it may not be possible in the existing environment, the ministry and the TB program should consider setting up a health technology assessment unit for providing input in such decision-making. This will ensure that decisions are evidence-informed and not unduly influenced by the priorities and perception of powerful stakeholders.

References

1. Mitnick C, Bayona J, Palacios E, et al. Community-based therapy for multidrug-resistant tuberculosis in Lima, Peru. *N Engl J Med.* 2003;348(2):119–128. doi: 10/fsh4rd
2. World Health Organization. *WHO Operational Handbook on Tuberculosis: Module 4: Treatment: Drug-Resistant Tuberculosis Treatment.* World Health Organization; 2020. Accessed October 1, 2021. https://apps.who.int/iris/handle/10665/332398

3. Mitnick CD, Shin SS, Seung KJ, et al. Comprehensive treatment of extensively drug-resistant tuberculosis. *N Engl J Med.* 2008;359(6):563–574. doi: 10.1056/ NEJMoa0800106

4. Drobac PC, Mukherjee JS, Joseph JK, et al. Community-based therapy for children with multidrug-resistant tuberculosis. *Pediatrics.* 2006;117(6):2022–2029. doi: 10.1542/peds.2005-2235

5. Furin JJ, Mitnick CD, Shin SS, et al. Occurrence of serious adverse effects in patients receiving community-based therapy for multidrug-resistant tuberculosis. *Int J Tuberc Lung Dis.* 2001;5(7):648–655.

6. Shin S, Furin J, Bayona J, Mate K, Kim JY, Farmer P. Community-based treatment of multidrug-resistant tuberculosis in Lima, Peru: 7 years of experience. *Soc Sci Med.* 2004;59(7):1529–1539. doi: 10.1016/j.socscimed.2004.01.027

7. Keshavjee S, Farmer PE. Tuberculosis, drug resistance, and the history of modern medicine. *N Engl J Med.* 2012;367(10):931–936. doi: 10.1056/NEJMra1205429

8. Kim JY, Mukherjee JS, Rich ML, Mate K, Bayona J, Becerra MC. From multidrug-resistant tuberculosis to DOTS expansion and beyond: Making the most of a paradigm shift. *Tuberculosis.* 2003;83(1):59–65. doi: 10.1016/S1472-9792(02)00078-1

9

Does Home-Based Neonatal Care of Sepsis Improve Neonatal Mortality?

RACHEL LUSK

> Reasons for the high acceptance of home-based care were: the huge unmet need of neonatal care in villages, involvement of traditional birth attendants, health education, good quality of care, availability of care at home by a village health worker resident in the village, successful management of sepsis, the faith of rural people in injections, and good motivation, training, supervision and performance-linked remuneration for the village health workers.[1]
>
> —BANG ET AL.

Research Question: Can home-based interventions for neonatal sepsis decrease neonatal mortality in developing countries where access to a hospital for these services is limited?

Funding: The Ford Foundation, USA, and the John D. and Catherine T. MacArthur Foundation, USA, supported the study financially. The protocol development phase was supported by a grant from the International Women's Health Coalition, New York.

Year Study Began: April 1993

Year Study Ended: March 1998

Location: Villages in Gadchiroli District, India (Maharashtra state)

Who Was Studied: Neonates born in 86 villages participating in the study (39 intervention and 47 control villages).

Who Was Excluded: Fourteen villages were excluded from the study due to a population of less than 300 people, or they were unable to find women in the village who could be trained to act as a village health worker.

How Many Patients: 10,191

Study Overview: See Figure 9.1.

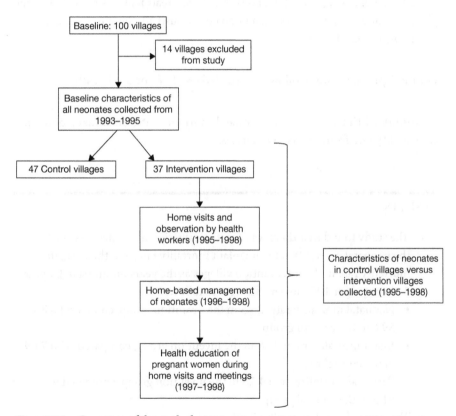

Figure 9.1. Overview of the study design.

Study Intervention: A census and baseline survey were performed in the research villages in 1993. Baseline data were collected on live births, neonatal deaths, and infant deaths from April 1993 to March 1995. A female social worker did unstructured interviews and observation of neonatal care at home to help plan the content of health education.

Village women who met specific criteria were chosen as village health workers and underwent 6 months of training. In-home neonatal care was then introduced in those 39 villages. Village health workers collected information on pregnant women and neonates, as well as provided protocolized care for minor illnesses and pneumonia in the neonates. In the second year of the study the village workers underwent additional training in management of neonatal sepsis with protocolized diagnosis and treatment and began offering at-home care if parents refused hospitalization. In the third year the village workers added health education to their home visits.

Of note, a physician visited each village once every 2 weeks to verify the data and educate the village health workers. No direct treatment was provided by the physician; however, if they found a neonate seriously ill, the physician again advised hospital admission.

Follow-Up: Infants were followed until 28 days of life, or until death.

Endpoints: Primary outcome: neonatal mortality rate. Secondary outcome: case fatality rate from sepsis in neonates.

RESULTS

- The study found that there was a statistically significant decrease in the neonatal mortality rate, the infant mortality rate, and the perinatal mortality rate in the intervention villages as the years progressed. By year 3, the rates per 1000 live births were as follows:
  - Neonatal mortality rate: 25.5 in the invention group, compared with 59.6 in the control group
  - Infant mortality rate: 38.8 in the invention group, compared with 74.9 in the control group
  - Perinatal mortality rate: 47.8 in the invention group, compared with 91.5 in the control group.
- There was also a statistically significant decrease in case fatality in neonatal sepsis, from 16.6% to 2.8% after treatment by village health workers.
- In the last year of the study, home-based neonatal care averted 1 death for every 18 neonates cared for.

Criticisms and Limitations:

- The definition of sepsis that is used is broad and nonspecific, making it possible that there were overdiagnosis and treatment in infants that did not actually have sepsis.
- There was no decrease in the proportion of neonates in the intervention area that were admitted to the hospital over the 3 years; however, it is possible that as word travels that in-home village health worker care is an option, it may detrimentally affect parents' willingness to take their children to the hospital for severe illness.
- The study points out that every family was advised to seek care at a hospital before home-based care was presented as another option. This study raises ethical concerns in that if a hospital exists that can treat a seriously ill infant, it may not be ethical to instead offer care by a community health worker and to not focus efforts on reducing barriers to access.
- The biggest risk of misinterpreting this study is that it unburdens the public health systems of their responsibility to set up newborn intensive care unit and care facilities.

Other Relevant Studies and Information:

- Since this study was published, there have been many governmental initiatives and programs that look at increasing access to neonatal care in India.
- The National Rural Health Mission (NRHM) was established in 2005. Under the NRHM, there was a linking of community- and facility-based care, as well as referrals between various levels of the healthcare system. As part of this, Special Newborn Care Units (SNCUs) were established for sick babies which provide level II care, allowing for those infants not requiring ventilators or surgery to be cared for closer to home in more rural districts.[2]
- Other programs and strategies have also been used to promote childbirth in facilities, including free transportation, care, medicines, and diagnostics in all public facilities.[3]

Summary and Implications: This study demonstrated that in areas where access to hospital-based neonatal care is limited, home-based interventions involving female village health workers can favorably impact case fatality from sepsis as well as the overall neonatal mortality rate.

PUBLIC HEALTH CASE: INCREASING ACCESS TO CARE

Case Overview

You are part of the Ministry of Health in Chhattisgarh, India. The hospital staff are typically not from the villages they serve. The villagers tend to be very traditional and are skeptical of hospitals and healthcare and do not always utilize the services available to them. You are asked to identify ways to increase access to healthcare in these regions. Drawing from the examples discussed in this chapter and other chapters, what might you suggest?

Suggested Answer

To address the barriers to care in these areas, it would be prudent to build relationships with the communities you are attempting to address in order to understand more about their priorities and needs and to gain trust. You should investigate the biggest health issues facing those communities. Performing a community needs assessment and interviewing local leaders about the communities' concerns, traditional values and beliefs, and perceptions of the healthcare they currently receive would be an important step.

With this information, you can evaluate ways to incorporate the community into their own care to promote trust, such as through a community or village health worker. Similar to this study, if patients are unwilling to go to a hospital and it is unfeasible to have hospital staff doing home visits, it may be possible to use community health workers or volunteer health workers to provide protocolized in-home treatment for certain illnesses or conditions. Additionally, consider other ways to reduce barriers to healthcare access: reducing or eliminating fees, providing food to patients and caregivers while hospitalized, improving roads, access to reliable transportation, and setting up clinics or smaller hospitals that are closer to home for patients, such as the SNCUs mentioned above.

References

1. Bang AT, Bang RA, Baitule SB, Reddy MH, Deshmukh MD. Effect of home-based neonatal care and management of sepsis on neonatal mortality: Field trial in rural India. *Lancet.* 1999;354(9194):1955–1961.
2. Neogi SB, Malhotra S, Zodpey S, Mohan P. Assessment of special care newborn units in India. *J Health Popul Nutr.* 2011;29(5):500.
3. Paul VK, Kumar R, Zodpey S. Toward single digit neonatal mortality rate in India. *J Perinatol.* 2016;36(s3):S1–S2.

SECTION 2

Social Medicine and Ethics

❝Martin Luther King Jr. remarked: "Of all the forms of inequality, injustice in healthcare is the most shocking and the most inhumane." Section 2, Social Medicine and Ethics—arguably the most important section in this book and a worthy read as an entire book on its own—takes care to include studies demonstrating injustice in healthcare and the impact of socioeconomic class, gender, nutrition, race, and power in the health of populations.

This section includes landmark studies that help form the basis of the argument for the social determinants of health, including the Barker Hypothesis, Whitehall studies, and the Papworth experiment".

10

Early Life Deprivation and Developmental Origins of Adult Metabolic Disease

Thrifty Phenotype Hypothesis/Barker Hypothesis

BASSEM GHALI

Processes linked to growth and acting in prenatal or early postnatal life strongly influence risk of ischaemic heart disease.

—BARKER ET AL.[1]

Research Question: Is there an association between birthweight, weight at 1 year, and mortality from ischemic heart disease in adults?

Funding: Records preserved by Hertfordshire County Archives; University of Southampton Archives, which stored the records during data abstraction. Staff at the National Health Service Central Register (NHSCR), Southport, and Office of Population Censuses and Surveys (OPCS), London, traced the men. The Milk Marketing Board gave a grant to assist tracing.

Year Study Began: 1951

Year Study Published: 1989

Study Location: Six registration districts in East Hertfordshire, United Kingdom

Who Was Studied: Adult men who were born 1911–1930 in the 6 registration districts.

Who Was Excluded: Those who died in childhood, came from twins/triplet pregnancies (only singleton births included), without birth weight or weight at 1 year, without enough data to query the NHS central registry, and those who were unable to be traced.

How Many Participants: 5654

Study Overview: Retrospective, observational cohort study (see Figure 10.1).

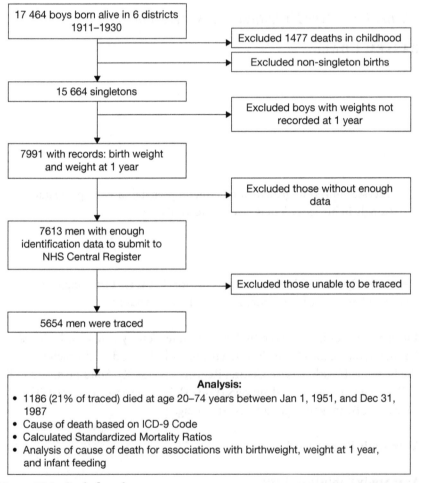

Figure 10.1. Study flow sheet.

Study Intervention: Cause of death and standardized mortality ratios were assessed for this population cohort of men, born between 1911 to 1930, based on birth weight, weight at 1 year, and feeding method.

Follow-Up: 57 to 78 years

Endpoints: Standardized mortality ratio (SMR) of ischemic heart disease, chronic obstructive pulmonary disease (COPD), lung cancer, and death from all causes analyzed with respect to birth weight, weight at 1 year, and feeding method.

RESULTS

- Babies with low birthweight (<5.5 pounds) had higher SMR of ischemic heart disease, COPD, and death from all causes. This was not observed for lung cancer.
- Infants who weighed more at 1 year of age were significantly less likely to die of ischemic heart disease. Among those who weighed 17 lb (7.7 kg) or less at 1 year, death rate from ischemic heart disease was 3 times greater than those who weighed 27 lb (12.2 kg) or more at 1 year. This was also noted in deaths from all causes.
- Men who weighed 5.5 lb (2.5 kg) or less at birth had the highest SMR for ischemic heart disease, but there was no significant downward trend in SMR for ischemic heart disease as birth weight increased. These men also had a higher risk of death from COPD and from all causes combined.
- Among those who died, mean birthweight and mean weight at 1 year did not differ among the 5 social classes.

Criticisms and Limitations:

- The study only examined men in a cohort born almost 100 years ago in the United Kingdom, perhaps limiting the generalizability to a more modern and global society.
- Study did not include data on gestational age, although we expect survival of a significant number of preterm babies only in recent medical history.[2] If, and by how much, prematurity contributes to the effect of low birth weight on ischemic heart disease later in life is unknown, but some studies suggest prematurity itself is a risk factor.[2]
- The epidemiological associations identified in this analysis may not represent a causal relationship.[5] The study also did not explicitly control for possible confounders such as socioeconomic status that may have explained the observed associations.

Other Relevant Studies and Information:

- The association between low birthweight and increased coronary artery disease has been observed in other analyses, as has an association with other cardiovascular and metabolic diseases and in different countries.[1–3] It is hypothesized that programming in fetal development is the underlying phenomenon driving this association, with several triggers such as fetal nutrition or increased glucocorticoid exposure.[2]
- The "thrifty phenotype" hypothesis proposes that poor fetal and infant nutrition leads to fetal glucose-conserving adaptations, which persist into adulthood and are linked with insulin resistance.[1,2]
- Epigenetic imprinting is thought to be the mechanism that links the intrauterine environment to altered gene expression and susceptibility to chronic disease in adulthood.[2,4]

Summary and Implications: This study demonstrates that low birthweight and low weight at 1 year of age pose a 3-fold increased risk of death from ischemic heart disease later in life. This suggests that targeted social programs that alleviate poverty and food scarcity to address the social determinants of health of women and their infants will reduce deaths from ischemic heart disease in the future. Of note, these findings show an epidemiologic correlation but do not prove causality.

CLINICAL CASE: THINKING ABOUT EARLY LIFE EVENTS AND THE EFFECTS ON FUTURE HEALTH

Case History

Jan Swasthya Sahyog is a secondary care hospital in Ganiyari, a rural district in Chhattisgarh, a state in central India. It serves a largely destitute population of people from marginalized castes and shunned Indigenous tribes who come from a wide encatchment area of rural districts and villages in the tiger reserve forests. There are high rates of communicable diseases like tuberculosis and diseases of poverty like severe malnutrition, but a paradoxically high rate of diabetes mellitus. An interesting subset of these patients, in their twenties and thirties, presented with lean diabetes that emerged in young adulthood, without clear ketoacidosis, and had a very low body mass index. This particular phenotype was discordant with the type 2 diabetes described in more urban areas, or in Western societies where patients with diabetes are often overweight. Utilizing the concepts presented by the Barker hypothesis, what social determinants of health may have contributed to this phenotype?

Suggested Answer

The etiology of lean diabetes has been debated, but one theory that has been proposed parallels the Barker hypothesis: that early life environmental influences (including in utero factors) may be risk factors for development of metabolic diseases such as diabetes, or in Barker's study ischemic heart disease. The importance of Barker's study and the possible connection with illnesses like lean diabetes highlight several important concepts. Social determinants of health that negatively impact maternal health may increase the risk of diseases in the next generation, akin to genetic mutation. Importantly, this raises the possibility that improving the living conditions, working conditions, and lives of people today not only improves their health, but also may work to prevent a significant burden of chronic diseases in future generations.

References

1. Barker DJ, Winter PD, Osmond C, Margetts B, Simmonds SJ. Weight in infancy and death from ischaemic heart disease. *Lancet.* 1989;2(8663):577–580.
2. Boo HA de, Harding JE. The developmental origins of adult disease (Barker) hypothesis. *Australian NZJ Obstet Gynaecol.* 2006;46(1):4–14.
3. Hales CN, Barker DJ. The thrifty phenotype hypothesis. *Br Med Bull.* 2001;60:5–20.
4. Young LE. Imprinting of genes and the Barker hypothesis. *Twin Res.* 2001;4(5):307–317.
5. Skogen JC, Overland S. The fetal origins of adult disease: A narrative review of the epidemiological literature. *JRSM Short Rep.* 2012;3(8):59.

11

Gender Disparity and Heart Diseases in South Africa

ABHISAKE KOLE

> Currently, [cardiovascular disease] is not being optimally managed in this rural area of South Africa. . . . Efforts to improve secondary prevention in this population should be focused on females, subjects from lower socioeconomic status, and those with physical disabilities.
>
> —JARDIM ET AL.[1]

Research Question: What are the patient characteristics associated with control of risk factors to prevent secondary cardiovascular disease in rural South Africa?

Funding: National Institute on Aging, National Institutes of Health, USA; University of Witwatersrand, South Africa; Medical Research Council, UK; Wellcome Trust, UK

Year Study Began: November 2014

Year Study Ended: November 2015

Year Study Published: 2017

Study Location: Agincourt subdistrict of Mpumalanga province in rural South Africa

Who Was Studied: All adults over 40 years of age, who had permanently resided in the Agincourt subdistrict for at least 1 year, were eligible. From this larger group, a subset with prior cardiovascular disease (CVD), defined by self-history of prior stroke or myocardial infarction or angina diagnosed by the Rose criteria,[2] was identified.

Who Was Excluded: People younger than 40, those who lived in Agincourt district for less than 1 year, and those who moved or died prior to study recruitment were excluded.

How Many Patients: 5059

Study Overview: The number of cardiovascular risk factors controlled among people with a history of CVD was analyzed as a function of biological, social, and economic factors (Figure 11.1).

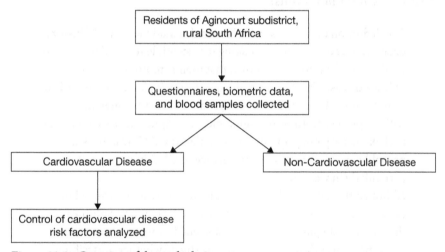

Figure 11.1. Overview of the study design.

Study Intervention: This was a cohort study that examined control of risk factors associated with cardiovascular disease. It collected socioeconomic data, anthropometric data, and clinical data including blood pressure, human immunodeficiency virus status, point-of-care glucose and lipid levels.

Follow-Up: There was no follow-up period; rather, this study simply looked for epidemiologic correlations.

Endpoints: Effective control of the following cardiovascular risk factors: (low-density lipoprotein cholesterol <1.8 mmol/L, blood pressure <140/90, smoking cessation, waist-to-hip ratio <0.9 for men or <0.85 for women, and body mass index <25 kg/m^2).

RESULTS

- 592/5059 (11.7%) of people had CVD; 62.2% of those with CVD were women, significantly higher than 53.6% of women in the study overall.
- 55.8% of men had 3 or more risk factors under control, compared to only 34.2% of women (p <0.001).
- Absence of physical disability and higher socioeconomic status were also associated with more cardiovascular risk factors controlled.
- Age, HIV status, immigrant status, or literacy were not associated with the number of risk factors controlled.

Criticisms and Limitations:

- The definition of "established" CVD in this study was by self-history or self-report of symptoms, making it susceptible to recall bias. Study participants may not have known that their symptoms were indicative of heart disease. Furthermore, the questionnaire focused primarily on symptoms of chest pain. Women are more likely than men to present with atypical symptoms of angina such as dyspnea, nausea, vomiting, back pain, jaw pain, palpitations, or indigestion.[3,4] Thus, this study probably underestimates the prevalence of CVD in its population, particularly in women.
- Although the authors identify a gender disparity in the control of cardiovascular risk factors in people with CVD in rural South Africa, they do not adequately discuss the societal factors that led to this outcome. The authors also did not investigate whether prescribing practices by healthcare providers contributed to the gender disparity seen in secondary prevention of CVD.
- Finally, the authors extrapolate their results in rural South Africa to the whole of sub-Saharan Africa (SSA). SSA is a heterogeneous area with diverse populations and cultural norms. Thus, the authors should be careful to apply their results only within the context they studied.

Other Relevant Studies and Information:

- In England, women with CVD were less likely to be prescribed statins or aspirin than men, even though they had higher LDL cholesterol levels and no contraindications to aspirin.[5]

- Mortality after myocardial infarction is higher in women than in men, particularly for ST elevation myocardial infarction[6] and those less than 75 years old.[7] Compared to men, women had a delayed presentation to the hospital, delayed diagnosis, and lower rates of reperfusion therapy.[7,8]
- In India, less money is spent on healthcare for women, even though women have higher rates of short-term and major morbidity from illness compared to men.[9]

Summary and Implications: Women with CVD have worse control of cardio-vascular risk factors compared to men in rural South Africa. This gender disparity extends beyond South Africa, including regions with variable socioeconomic status.

CLINICAL CASE: ADDRESSING GENDER DISPARITY IN MEDICAL CARE

Case History

You are working at a rural primary care clinic in a low- to middle-income country (LMIC). You have noticed that there is poor control of cardiovas-cular risk factors in patients with known CVD. You would like to improve the quality of secondary prevention of CVD at your clinic. What factors should you keep in mind and how does that guide your approach?

Suggested Answer

This study and others have identified a gender disparity in the treatment of CVD. Thus, one must be cognizant of poorer control of cardiovascular risk factors in women when addressing secondary prevention of CVD and take actionable measures to bridge the gap. Women will likely need more coun-seling at the time of primary diagnosis of their CVD to emphasize that heart disease can affect women as much as men and to make them aware of atyp-ical symptoms. Because many societies are patriarchal, this counseling may be best if it involves the entire family, including male members as part of the care team. At the time of diagnosis, a close follow-up date should be set. If the patient does not show up to their follow-up, the reasons why must be investigated. Some possible barriers to seeking care may be household duties, care for other family members, transportation, or the cost of health-care. Identifying these barriers can help in creating plans to achieve greater gender equity.

References

1. Jardim TV, et al. Disparities in management of cardiovascular disease in rural South Africa: Data from the HAALSI (Health and Aging in Africa: Longitudinal Studies of INDEPTH Communities) Study. *Circ Cardiovasc Qual Outcomes*. 2017 Nov;10(11):e004094.
2. Achterberg S, et al. Prognostic value of the Rose questionnaire: A validation with future coronary events in the SMART study. *Eur J Prev Cardiol*. 2012 Feb;19(1):5–14.
3. Dey S, et al. Sex-related differences in the presentation, treatment and outcomes among patients with acute coronary syndromes: The Global Registry of Acute Coronary Events. *Heart*. 2009 Jan;95(1):20–26. doi: 10.1136/hrt.2007.138537.
4. Milner KA, et al. Gender differences in symptom presentation associated with coronary heart disease. *Am J Cardiol*. 1999 Aug 15;84(4):396–399.
5. Hippisley-Cox J, et al. Sex inequalities in ischaemic heart disease in general practice: cross sectional survey. *BMJ*. 2001 Apr 7;322(7290):832.
6. Berger JS, et al. Sex differences in mortality following acute coronary syndromes. *JAMA*. 2009;302(8):874–882. doi:10.1001/jama.2009.1227
7. Vaccarino V, et al. Sex-based differences in early mortality after myocardial infarction. *N Engl J Med*. 1999;341:217–22.5
8. Barron HV, Bowlby LJ, Breen T, et al. Use of reperfusion therapy for acute myocardial infarction in the United States: Data from the National Registry of Myocardial Infarction 2. *Circulation*. 1998;97:1150–1156.
9. Saikia N, et al. Gender difference in health-care expenditure: Evidence from India Human Development Survey. *PLoS One*. 2016;11(7):e0158332.

12

Economic Growth and Child Undernourishment

ARKAPRABHA GUN

We failed to find consistent evidence that economic growth leads to reduction in childhood undernutrition in India. Direct investments in appropriate health interventions may be necessary to reduce childhood
undernutrition in India.

—SUBRAMANYAM ET AL.[1]

Research Question: Does observational evidence show that macroeconomic
growth leads to a reduction in child undernutrition in India?

Years Studied: 1992–2005

Year Study Published: 2011

Study Location: India

Units of Observation for Data: Repeated cross-sectional data made available through three different rounds of the National Family Health Survey
(NFHS): 1992–1993, 1998–1999, and 2005–2006.

What Was Studied: The effect of macroeconomic growth, data on which were
made available by the Reserve Bank of India, on child health indicators made
available through the three different rounds of the NFHS.

What Units of Observation Were Excluded: The states of Tripura and Sikkim, due to the absence of information on child health indicators in the 1998–1999, and 1992–1993 rounds of the NFHS. Observations with missing data on covariates that were included in the estimated regressions were also excluded.

Sample Size of Data Used: After excluding data on missing states and records with missing data on covariates, a final sample size of 77 326, 56 774, and 56 721 were used for the analyses of underweight, stunting, and wasting, respectively.

Study Overview: The study uses secondary data made available for India to study possible linkages between macroeconomic growth and reduction in child undernourishment, over the period 1992–2005 (see Figure 12.1). The study uses definitions standardized by the World Health Organization to classify a child's nourishment level by calculating Z-scores for the anthropomorphic indicators. The statistical model estimated is in the form of a multilevel logistic regression. This particular kind of logistic regression allows one to account for the clustering of subjects within a higher-level unit (e.g., in this case the higher-level unit is the state, an administrative unit made up of individuals). This allowed the author to estimate the effect that state-level economic growth can have on an individual's chance of experiencing different nourishment outcomes (stunting, wasting, or being underweight).

RESULTS

- The authors estimated the odds ratio of the children being underweight, stunted, or suffering from wasting, given a 5000 Indian rupees (INR) increase in the state per capita income. Across all three outcomes, the OR and confidence interval of the estimated OR had values of around 1.00, including the confidence interval. This implies that the likelihood of a child experiencing undernourishment does not vary in a statistically significant manner, as a result of state-level economic growth.
- The results were the same in the cases for severe undernutrition outcomes, except that of stunting. In this case, an increase in 5000 INR over 6.5 years seems to have led to a marginally higher, but statistically significant increase in the risk of suffering from severe stunting.
- The associations between undernutrition and social factors like wealth were as expected, with children from the lowest stratum of society having a significantly higher risk of being underweight, stunted, or wasted. The effect of not having parents who attended school was similarly high and significant on the risk of being undernourished, with the estimated risk of

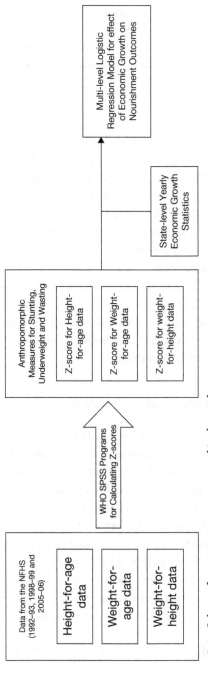

Figure 12.1. Schema for estimation strategy used in the study.

being undernourished twice as high for children who did not have school-educated parents.

- This resulted in the authors concluding that there was no empirical evidence in the Indian context that reflected the macroeconomic growth that led to a significantly lower risk of suffering from undernutrition.

Criticisms and Limitations:

- As the authors themselves have noted, this study has had the problem of suffering from missing data for a significant number of observations. To counter this problem, the authors ran a variety of estimation exercises to get around this limitation. This includes running estimations for years without missing data, and the estimates generated were not significantly different from the ones with missing data. Thus, the estimates of the study itself would be considered to be relatively free from bias.
- Another limitation that the authors have noted is that the condition of economic well-being was measured using the household wealth or asset index. This index is difficult to interpret in absolute terms, and the authors were unable to test whether state-level macroeconomic growth increased household wealth levels.

Other Relevant Studies and Information:

- "Health and Economic Growth" (2018), by Bloom, Kuhn, and Prettner,[2] discusses the macroeconomic effects of disease and epidemics. They conduct a review of how economic consequences depend on the characteristics of the disease and preexisting inequalities.
- "The Reversal of the Relation between Economic Growth and Health Progress: Sweden in the 19th and 20th Centuries" (2018), by Granados and Ionides,[3] examines the case of Sweden, where the relationship between economic growth and health progress was negative in the 19th century and was subsequently reversed in the 20th century. The study tries to discuss why this must be the case and re-emphasizes that economic growth does not guarantee better health outcomes.

Summary and Implications: This study examines the effect that state-level economic growth has on nutritional outcomes in children. This paper is innovative in that it uses a multilevel model, which allows the authors to estimate how an aggregate outcome (growth) can affect the individual risk of undernourishment. The analysis failed to identify a correlation between state-level economic growth over a period of 15 years (1992–2006) with the risk of undernourishment. Hence, a more targeted policy may be required to ensure that increase in national incomes translates to improved nutritional outcomes for children.

POLICY CASE STUDY: ECONOMIC GROWTH INCENTIVES OR TARGETED CHILD NUTRITION POLICIES?

Case History

You have been approached by a health official for a district in India for advice. The latest round of the NFHS data has shown a worsening outcome for the district in terms of anthropomorphic indicators for nutrition. The official feels that the current COVID-19 pandemic has contributed to this phenomenon through the economic fallout that was generated. Do you advise them to spend their discretionary budget on economic growth incentivizing policy—or on targeted schemes like the Integrated Child Development Scheme (ICDS)?

Suggested Answer

While the source of the sliding indicators of child nutrition may be due to worsening economic outlook, focusing simply on the economic element may not be enough to solve the nutrition crisis, as this paper demonstrates. It is advisable to direct the official to spend their discretionary budget on ensuring that preexisting schemes like the mid-day meal system are functioning, maybe by delivering unused food grain to the households during the time that schools remain closed due to pandemic restrictions.

Mid-day meals have been effective in both incentivizing enrollment and improving nutritional outcomes. They are a part of the ICDS mentioned previously, and spending money on increasing the outreach of the program may be more effective than incentivizing economic growth. This is more important given that the growth in incomes may be unequal and the underserved may not necessarily experience the benefits of growth.

Another challenge regarding economic policies not specific to nutrition is that families might invest additional income on quasi-luxury items such as motorcycles and not on a more balanced diet.

References

1. Subramanyam MA, Kawachi I, Berkman LF, Subramanian SV. Is economic growth associated with reduction in child undernutrition in India? *PLoS Med.* 2011;8(3):e1000424. doi:10.1371/journal.pmed.1000424
2. Bloom DE, Kuhn M, Prettner K. Health and economic growth. Oxford Research Encyclopedia of Economics and Finance. Retrieved 20 July, 2020, from https://oxfor dre.com/economics/view/10.1093/acrefore/9780190625979.001.0001/acrefore-9780190625979-e-36.
3. Tapia Granados JA, Ionides EL. The reversal of the relation between economic growth and health progress: Sweden in the 19th and 20th centuries. *J Health Econ.* 2008;27(3):544–563. doi:10.1016/j.jhealeco.2007.09.006

13

Can Social Interventions Prevent Tuberculosis?

The Papworth Experiment (1918–1943) Revisited

ERICA TATE

Results indicate that conditions at Papworth did not reduce the risk of tuberculosis (TB) infection. . . . Rather, the Papworth experiment was associated with a substantially reduced risk of disease and related deaths.[1]

Research Question: Do social interventions reduce tuberculosis (TB) transmission or incidence of disease in child household contacts of patients with TB?

Funding: Grants from the European Commission (TBSusgent) and the EDCTP (TB-NEAT)

Year Study Began: Papworth Study, 1918–1943; Papworth Study Revisited, 2012

Year Study Published: 2012

Study Location: Papworth Village Settlement, England

Who Was Studied: The analysis focused on 315 children who lived with a parent with active TB at the Papworth Village Settlement during the years 1918–1943.

Who Was Excluded: Children of families admitted to Papworth that never resided at Papworth, as well as the children of healthy staff members living in the Papworth Village.

How Many Patients: 315

Study Overview: See Figure 13.1.

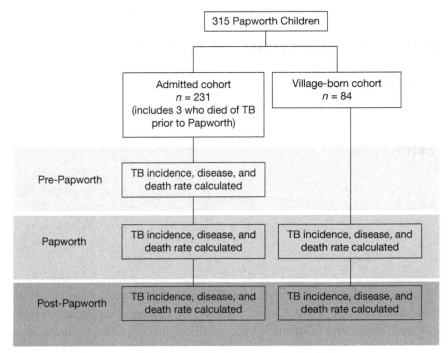

Figure 13.1. Summary of the Papworth Experiment revisited design.

Study Intervention: The Papworth Village Settlement provided comprehensive social support in the form of housing, adequate nutrition, healthcare, and employment for patients with TB and their families after their discharge from a sanatorium. In 1937, a survey was conducted to document the outcomes of TB infection and disease in children in the Settlement during 1918–1938. The status of children was updated until 1943.

In this study, the authors abstracted data from the original study. They separated the children into two broad cohorts: village-born (born in Papworth after their parents were admitted) and admitted cohort (brought to Papworth with their families after release from a sanatorium). Infection rates in children were analyzed at discrete time periods: pre-Papworth (children evaluated prior to their admission to Papworth), Papworth (village-born or admitted cohort children while living within the Settlement), and post-Papworth periods (either village-born or admitted children after leaving the Settlement).

Follow-Up: Until the child left Papworth or the end of the study (median 6.5–9 years)

Endpoints: Primary endpoints pertained to possible childhood disease burden:
- Normal: no clinical or radiologic abnormalities to suggest TB infection or disease
- TB infection: absence of symptoms, but some abnormal radiographic findings (i.e., Ghon focus, calcified foci, transient radiographic densities)
- TB disease: presence of clinical symptoms of TB with sputum smear and gastric lavage positive or radiologic abnormalities on serial x-rays.

RESULTS

- Annual TB infection incidence rate was similar between both cohorts while living in Papworth: 20% for village-born children and 24% for admitted cohorts (Table 13.1).
- Among children 5 years of age or less, there was zero incidence of TB in the village-born group compared with five cases among children born outside Papworth (Table 13.1).
- Among children admitted to Papworth who were 13 years and older, the risk of TB before admission to Papworth was 5263/100 000 person-years, whereas it was 341/100 000 person-years while living in Papworth.
- Post-Papworth the incidence rates appeared to rise again: in the 13-year and older group, incidence of TB was 2439/100 000 person years after discharge from Papworth.

Table 13.1 SUMMARY OF PAPWORTH REVISITED'S KEY FINDINGS

	Pre-Papworth Admitted	Papworth Village-born	Admitted	Post-Papworth Village-born	Admitted
Morbidity*	8	1	5	0	5
Mortality	6	0	2	0	4
Incidence rate of TB					
Age group <5	1,217	0	0	0	0
Age group 6–12	578	330	131	0	0
Age group >13	5263	0	341	0	2439

* Children with TB disease

Criticisms and Limitations: The follow-up for the admitted and village-born children was limited. Only 34 children from the admitted cohort returned to the settlement for evaluation and only 3 from the village-born cohort returned. Follow-up was lacking for significant comparison of the TB outcomes post-Papworth.

Other Relevant Studies and Information:

- Malnutrition has been associated with increased incidence of TB in children and decreased efficacy of BCG vaccination. Malnutrition increases the risk of active disease and poor outcomes of TB treatment. In the review article "Undernutrition and Tuberculosis in India: Situation Analysis and the Way Forward," data supporting nutritional support for those at risk for TB infection and the need for these interventions in India are outlined.[3]
- A recent Peruvian study also supports directed social interventions to improve TB treatment outcomes. The authors evaluated outcomes concerning enrollment in preventive TB therapy and treatment to cure among members of households with a positive TB contact. The authors provided cash transfers in a resource-constrained population which decreased the catastrophic costs of treatment for families, and led to improved outcomes and higher rates of cure.[5]

Summary and Implications: The Papworth experiment was an early example of the importance of social factors such as housing, nutrition, and access to medical care, in decreasing TB disease and death rates in close contact household members. Decades later, the need for these types of interventions in TB care are still being discussed. There is recognition that poverty and income inequality are correlated with TB rates.[2] The World Health Assembly's new End TB Strategy focuses on addressing social interventions to help combat the world TB infection and disease rates.[4] These interventions include programs like cash transfers, subsidized healthcare, housing subsidies, and food rations.[4]

CLINICAL CASE: SOCIAL DETERMINANTS IN TUBERCULOSIS

Case History

A 35-year-old Honduran male who immigrated to the United States last year presents with 2 months of cough and shortness of breath. He has been losing weight and endorses decreased energy level. He is concerned about his ability to work. He is the primary breadwinner for his family and his wife recently had a new baby. Chest x-ray (CXR) shows bilateral upper lobe infiltrates, sputum acid-fast Bacillus (AFB) smears are pending, and interferon gamma release assay returns positive.

What social factors will affect the quality of care for this patient and his family, and what potential barriers should you discuss and address?

Suggested Answer

As the sole source of income for his family, the course of hospitalization and treatment could create a large financial burden for this patient. Coordination of social support services such as supplemental food support and food banks may be needed. The importance of adequate nutrition for children and other family members should be discussed to attempt to reduce the rate of disease in household contacts. Costs such as family member testing, treatment, and transportation will need to be discussed and mitigated using local available resources.

References

1. Bhargava A, Pai M, Bhargava M, Marais BJ, Menzies D. Can social interventions prevent tuberculosis? The Papworth experiment (1918–1943) revisited. *Am J Resp Crit Care Med.* 2012;186(5):442–449. https://doi.org/10.1164/rccm.201201-0023OC.
2. Holtgrave DR, Crosby RA. Social determinants of tuberculosis case rates in the United States. *Am J Prev Med.* 2004;26(2):159–162. doi: 10.1016/j.amepre.2003.10.014
3. Padmapriyadarsini C, Shobana M, Lakshmi M, Beena T, Swaminathan S. Undernutrition and tuberculosis in India: Situation analysis and the way forward. *Indian J Med Res.* 2016;144(1):11–20. doi: 10.4103/0971-5916.193278
4. Siroka A, Ponce NA, Lönnroth K. Association between spending on social protection and tuberculosis burden: A global analysis. *Lancet Infect Dis.* 2016;16(4):473–479. doi: 10.1016/S1473-3099(15)00401-6
5. Wingfield T, Tovar MA, Huff D, et al. Beyond pills and tests: Addressing the social determinants of tuberculosis. *Clin Med (Lond).* 2016;16(Suppl 6):s79–s91. doi: 10.7861/clinmedicine.16-6-s79

14

Socioeconomic Status and Heart Disease

Whitehall Revisited

AMANDA BRADKE

> Were it possible to reduce the mortality rate of clerical officers in the civil service to that of administrators, they would have less than half their current death rate . . . [our data] suggest that attention should be paid to the social environment, job design, and the consequences of income inequality.
>
> —MARMOT ET AL.[1]

Research Question: To what degree does morbidity differ across social class (represented by employment grade) when assessed in a contemporary population that includes women, and what causes and factors could be contributing to this?

Funding: Information not found

Year Study Began: 1985

Year Study Published: 1991

Study Location: London, United Kingdom

Who Was Studied: Men and women civil-service workers, age 35–55 at the start of the study, who worked at 1 of 20 civil-service departments.

Who Was Excluded: Those who did not respond to the participation invite and those who moved before the study began.

How Many Patients: 10 314 (6900 men, 3414 women)

Study Overview: See Figure 14.1.

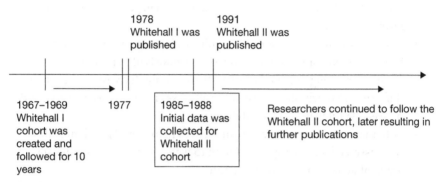

Figure 14.1. Overview of the study design.

Study Intervention:

Self-Administered Questionnaire: Extensive questionnaires were completed by participants and missing data were elicited during the examination. Topics covered include social and demographic data, health status measures (various previously validated symptom questionnaires and former formal diagnoses), work characteristics, social supports, health behaviors, locus of control, stressful life events, and personal difficulties.

Examination: Participants were asked to complete a screening examination with height and weight, blood pressure measurements, electrocardiogram (EKG), and a blood test for cholesterol levels. EKGs were coded by computer and, if labeled as possible or probable ischemia, were verified by an experienced human coder.

Follow-Up: Not mentioned explicitly; follow-up continues to date.

Endpoints:
- Prevalence of ischemic heart disease (based on angina symptoms, EKG findings) at the cross-sectional time point of the study intervention.
- Other morbidity indicators, such as self-rated health, health problems over the past year, and drug therapy for hypertension, were also included. All data were age-adjusted.

RESULTS

- The study found an inverse association between employment grade and prevalence of angina, EKG evidence of ischemia, and symptoms of bronchitis.
- Women were more likely to report symptoms of angina, despite having less evidence of ischemia by EKG criteria, with findings showing an inverse trend with employment grade. Women in general reported higher levels of morbidity.
- There was an inverse relationship with employment grade and self-rated health, diabetes, and for men, previous diagnosis of hypertension.
- When comparing matched cohorts, there was no decrease in the relative difference in morbidity between social classes in the 20-year time period between Whitehall I and Whitehall II.
- Potential factors to explain the differences in morbidity and mortality were assessed, and many were found to have a statistically significant gradient across employment grades:
  - Physiological differences: There was an inverse gradient between height and employment grade, with participants in the highest employment grade as the tallest. Participants in lower employment grades were more likely to be obese.
  - Social circumstance differences: Participants in lower employment grades demonstrated more financial and housing difficulties, more stressful life events, and for men, less satisfactory social support.
  - Behavioral differences: Participants with higher-status jobs reported higher leisure-time physical activities, indicators of healthy eating, and belief they could take action to prevent a heart attack. Higher employment grades reported higher alcohol consumption, while lower employment grades had higher rates of smoking.
  - Work environment differences: There was an inverse gradient between employment grade and likeliness to report control at work, use of skills, and work variety. Lower employment grades had lower job satisfaction.
- The statistically significant factors listed above showed a gradient across all employment grades, not just the worse outcomes clustered at the lowest-status employment grade.

Criticisms and Limitations:

- This study showed correlation between employment grade and factors that may help explain differences in morbidity and mortality; however, it was observational. A randomized trial would be necessary to demonstrate causation.
- Additionally, while each indicator was compared across employment grades, they were not assessed in relationship to each other.
- The study findings were less consistent among women vs. men.

Other Relevant Studies and Information:

- Whitehall I showed that persons working in the lowest UK civil servant employment grade were three times more likely to die from CHD than those who worked in the highest employment grade. This gradient was maintained, and largely unchanged, even after accounting for differences in obesity, cholesterol, smoking, blood pressure, blood glucose, physical activity, and height. In fact, employment grade, which represented social class, was found to be the single strongest predictor of CHD death in the study.
- A report from the World Health Organization's Commission on Social Determinants of Health, titled "Closing the Gap in a Generation," recommends improving the conditions of daily life, the circumstances in which people are born, grow, live, work, and age. It also recommends tackling the inequitable distribution of power, money, and resources, and training the health workforce in social determinants of health.[2]

Summary and Implications: In this cohort of stably employed civil servants, there was a clear gradient in health outcomes based on civil service grade. These findings suggest that factors such as work and social environment, life stressors, and lack of, or perceived lack of, opportunity and control may significantly influence health. The Whitehall studies serve as a key foundation for our current understanding of the social determinants of health.

CLINICAL CASE: BRINGING UNIQUE SOCIAL DETERMINANTS OF HEALTH INTO THE CLINIC

Case History

A 50-year-old man presents for a new patient examination. He has a history of hypertension and depression, and a family history remarkable for a myocardial infarction in his brother at the age of 70. He sees a counselor for depression, but does not feel he has good social support outside of this. He is currently employed as a clerical office worker, assisting 3–4 other employees in completing their job tasks. He endorses smoking a pack of cigarettes daily for the past 20 years. Based on the Whitehall II study, what factors could be contributing to his risk for heart disease, as well as other morbidity and mortality? How will you counsel him on approaches to improving his health?

Suggested Answer

According to Whitehall II, "Healthy behaviors should be encouraged across the whole society; more attention should be paid to the social environments, job design, and the consequences of income inequality."[3] Heeding this advice, for our current patient our discussion and recommendations need to go beyond the classically recognized risk factors for developing cardiovascular disease.

While it will be necessary to address smoking cessation and risk attributable to family history, it will also be important to discuss his social situation. In this vignette we learn that our patient struggles with depression and feels he does not have good social support. We also learn that he is a subordinate to many at work, in a role where his tasks depend on the needs of others. Exploring possible approaches to improving social support in his life and discussing his frame of mind in regard to his work duties and how he might be able to gain a stronger sense of control will hopefully improve his cardiovascular health outcomes, and morbidity and mortality in general.

References

1. Marmot MG, Rose G, Shipley M, Hamilton PJ. Employment grade and coronary heart disease in British civil servants. *J Epidemiol Community Health*. 1978;32(4):244–249. https://doi.org/10.1136/jech.32.4.244

2. Marmot MG, Stansfeld S, Patel C, et al. Health inequalities among British civil servants: The Whitehall II Study. *Lancet.* 1991;337(8754):1387–1393. https://doi.org/10.1016/0140-6736(91)93068-k

3. CSDH. Closing the gap in a generation: Health equity through action on the social determinants of health. *Final Report of the Commission on Social Determinants of Health.* World Health Organization; 2008:1–33.

15

Implicit Bias in Pain Management

Manifestations in Patient Care

KUANG-NING HUANG AND CRISTINA RIVERA CARPENTER

> Hispanic patients with isolated long-bone fractures are twice as likely
> as non-Hispanic white patients to receive no pain medications in [the
> Emergency Department].
>
> —TODD ET AL.[1]

Research Question: Are Hispanic patients more likely than non-Hispanic white
patients to receive no analgesic while being treated in the Emergency Department
(ED) for isolated long-bone fractures?

Funding: Not stated

Year Study Began: 1990

Year Study Published: 1993

Study Location: UCLA Emergency Medicine Center, Los Angeles, CA, USA

Who Was Studied: Patients between the ages of 15 to 55 years who were evaluated in the ED for isolated long-bone fractures between the dates of January 1,
1990, and December 31, 1991.

Who Was Excluded: Patients whose injury occurred more than 6 hours prior
to presentation in the ED, those identified to have only a "possible fracture" or

chip fracture, and those who had co-occurring altered mentation or ethanol intoxication.

How Many Patients: 139

Study Overview: Figure 15.1 provides an overview of the study design. The study was a retrospective cohort review of patients with isolated long bone fractures who presented to the emergency room during the defined study period. They were separated by ethnicity, as noted in the chart, and then a chart review was performed to see if analgesia was given.

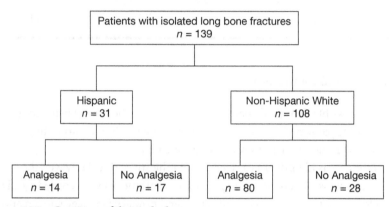

Figure 15.1. Overview of the study design.

Study Intervention: Not applicable.

Follow-Up: Completion of the ED stay

Endpoints: ED administration of analgesia or no analgesia

RESULTS

- 139 total patients met inclusion criteria for the study.
- 55% of Hispanic patients did not receive any analgesia, compared to 26% of non-Hispanic white patients, for the management of isolated long-bone extremity fractures. The relative risk (RR) of no analgesia was twice as great for Hispanic patients compared to non-Hispanic white patients in the study (Table 15.1).
- Controlling for covariates related to patient characteristics (sex, language, insurance status), severity of injury, physician characteristics, and potential

for association with ethanol intoxication did not result in substantial change in the study findings.
- Hispanic ethnicity was the strongest predictor of no analgesic administration.
- Of patients who received analgesia, Hispanic patients were more likely to receive oral analgesics, lower doses, or non-narcotic analgesia.

Table 15.1 SUMMARY OF KEY FINDINGS

	White, % (n)	Hispanic, % (n)	*p* Value
No analgesia	25.9 (28)	54.8 (17)	0.005
Low dose (<10 mg morphine)	45.4 (49)	19.4 (6)	0.005
High dose (>10 mg morphine)	28.7 (31)	25.8 (8)	0.005

Criticisms and Limitations:

- It is possible that the disparate use of analgesics between Hispanic vs. non-Hispanic patients is at least partially the result of confounding factors rather than entirely due to implicit bias.
- Ethnicity is identified as a risk factor in the study title. However, the data reviewed were based on *perception* of ethnic origin recorded by ED clerical staff on the basis of surnames and primary language spoken and not always patient self-identification.

Other Relevant Studies and Information:

- A meta-analysis of acute pain management in Emergency Departments demonstrated that Black and Hispanic patients are less likely to receive equivalent analgesia compared to non-Hispanic white patients.[2-6] Racial and ethnic disparities in pain management have been demonstrated across clinical settings,[3] such as outpatient care,[5] and in varying diagnostic conditions such as abdominal pain[6] and postpartum pain management.[2] These studies consistently demonstrate racial and ethnic minorities being at increased risk of receiving less-aggressive analgesia for management for similar diagnoses and/or pain scores compared to non-Hispanic white patients.
- Racial and socioeconomic disparities persist in healthcare.[7,8] The implicit bias surrounding race in this study could be extrapolated to other forms of implicit bias around gender, sexual identity or orientation, and socioeconomic status. Both care satisfaction and

provider trust are well-established predictors of numerous patient outcomes including medication adherence, healthcare utilization, and overall health status,[3] indicating that implicit bias may in this way directly result in the health disparities noted between varying population groups.

Summary and Implications: In this analysis of patients treated in the ED of a large academic medical center for long bone fractures, patients of Hispanic background were less likely to receive pain medication, and when they did receive opioid analgesia the dosage was lower. These findings suggest that implicit bias may affect medical decision-making.

CLINICAL CASE: A YOUNG WOMAN WITH ABDOMINAL PAIN

Case History
A young Navajo woman presents to the Emergency Department with sudden onset abdominal pain. This is her fourth visit to the ED in the past month for abdominal pain. Based on this study and the discussion on implicit bias, how do you see implicit bias potentially affecting her care?

Suggested Answer
- Implicit bias can lead to disparity in treatment modalities for patients presenting with similar diagnostic conditions. Potential downstream effects of minimized pain evaluation and treatment include undertreatment of pain, possible delay in diagnosis of urgent clinical concerns (e.g., appendicitis, ectopic pregnancy), and impact a patient's rapport with the healthcare system and potential willingness to re-engage in future care.
- Implicit bias is difficult to measure on an objective scale in studies. Bias is universal; awareness of bias is not. Bias does not suggest interpersonal conflict, nor does it describe intentions. A provider's own nationality or ethnic background does not preclude them from having implicit bias.
- Recognizing that implicit bias plays a role in patient care is important in order to break the cycle of attributing healthcare disparities solely to individual behaviors, biological differences, and cultural norms.

References

1. Todd KH, Samaroo N, Hoffman JR. Ethnicity as a risk factor for inadequate emergency department analgesia. *JAMA*. 1993;269(12):1537–1539. doi:10.1001/jama.1993.03500120075029
2. Badreldin N, Grobman WA, Yee LM. Racial disparities in postpartum pain management. *Obstet Gynecol*. 2019 Dec;134(6):1147–1153. doi: 10.1097/AOG.0000000000003561
3. Hall WJ, Chapman MV, Lee KM, et al. Implicit racial/ethnic bias among health care professionals and its influence on health care outcomes: A systematic review. *Am J Public Health*. 2015;105(12):e60–e76. doi:10.2105/AJPH.2015.302903
4. Lee P, Le Saux M, Siegel R, et al. Racial and ethnic disparities in the management of acute pain in US emergency departments: Meta-analysis and systematic review. *Am J Emerg Med*. 2019 Sep;37(9):1770–1777. doi: 10.1016/j.ajem.2019.06.014. PMID: 31186154.
5. Ly DP. Racial and ethnic disparities in the evaluation and management of pain in the outpatient setting, 2006–2015. *Pain Med*. 2019;20(2):223–232. doi: 10.1093/pm/pny074
6. Shah AA, Zogg CK, Zafar SN, et al. Analgesic access for acute abdominal pain in the emergency department among racial/ethnic minority patients: A nationwide examination. *Med Care*. 2015 Dec;53(12):1000–1009. doi: 10.1097/MLR.0000000000000444. PMID: 26569642.
7. National Academies of Sciences, Engineering, and Medicine; Health and Medicine Division; Board on Population Health and Public Health Practice; Committee on Community-Based Solutions to Promote Health Equity in the United States; Baciu A, Negussie Y, Geller A, et al., eds. *Communities in Action: Pathways to Health Equity*. Washington, DC: National Academies Press; 2017 Jan 11. 2, The State of Health Disparities in the United States. Available from: https://www.ncbi.nlm.nih.gov/books/NBK425844/
8. Chetty R, Stepner M, Abraham S, et al. The association between income and life expectancy in the United States, 2001–2014. *JAMA*. 2016;315(16):1750–1766. https://doi.org/10.1001/jama.2016.4226

16

Race-Based Medicine—Is It Biological or Profit Driven?

The African-American Heart Failure Trial (A-HeFT)

NADRA CRAWFORD

> The addition of a combination pill including isosorbide dinitrate (ISDN) and hydralazine with standard therapy improves survival in blacks with advanced heart disease over standard therapy alone.
>
> —TAYLOR ET AL.[1]

Research Question: Does the combination of isosorbide dinitrate (ISDN) and hydralazine improve survival in a single racial group with advanced heart failure over placebo?

Funding: NitroMed (pharmaceutical company)

Year study Began: 2001

Year Study Ended: 2004

Study Location: 161 sites throughout the USA

Who Was Included: Self-identifying Black men and women, 18 years and older who had a New York Heart Association (NYHA) class III/IV, who were receiving standard heart therapy treatment, and who had evidence of left ventricular dysfunction 6 months preceding the study.

Who Was Excluded: Pregnant women, nursing women, childbearing-aged women on less effective methods of contraception, all other racial groups, any patient with a contraindication to use of isosorbide dinitrate and/or hydralazine.

Number of Participants: 1050

Study Overview: Figure 16.1 provides an overview of the study design.

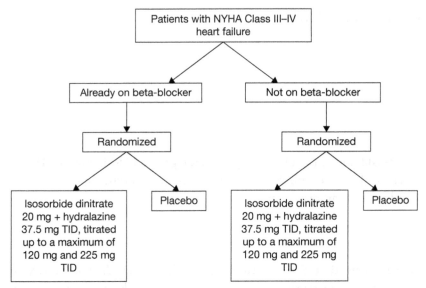

Figure 16.1. Summary of A-HeFT's design.

Study Intervention: Randomization was performed and groups were stratified according to background therapy with or without beta-blocker use. For each stratum there were blocks of 4 participants. Each site could randomize up to 6 blocks of non-beta-blocker users and 10 blocks of beta-blocker users. Participants were randomized into receiving a fixed dose combination ISDN and hydralazine or receiving placebo. Both groups continued with background therapy. Doses of ISDN and hydralazine started at 20 mg and 37.5 mg, respectively, 3 times per day (TID) and were titrated up to a maximum of 120 mg and 225 mg TID depending on absence of side effects.

Follow-Up: 10 months

Endpoints: All-cause mortality; a first hospitalization for heart failure during the 18 months; change in quality of life measured by a validated questionnaire.

RESULTS

- This study was stopped early based on a significantly higher mortality rate (10.2%) in the placebo group as compared to the treatment group (6.2%) ($p = 0.02$). There was a 43% improvement in survival in the treatment arm (Hazard ratio 0.57; $p = 0.01$ by the log bank test).
- There was a reduction in the rate of first hospitalization for heart failure (16.4% in the treatment arm and 24.4% in the placebo arm, $p = 0.001$)
- There was a statistically significant improvement in the mean primary composite score (consisting of rate of death from any cause, rate of first hospitalization from heart failure, and quality of life improvement) from –0.5 to –0.1 ($p = 0.01$) for the placebo group vs. treatment group, respectively.

Criticisms and Limitations:

- Based on the results of this analysis, it is unclear if hydralazine plus ISDN would provide benefits to other racial or ethnic groups.
- This study presupposes race as a discrete marker of biological difference instead of focusing on race as a social construct that results in health disparities and ignores non-genetic contributors of disease.[2,5] However, defenders of the FDA's decision note that this study did lead to approval of a drug that reduces mortality for an understudied population and may be an important, albeit imperfect, stepping stone in the progress of personalized medicine.

Similar Trials and Other Relevant Information:

- This study played an important role in the US Food and Drug Administration (FDA) approving ISDN/hydralazine specifically for African Americans with congestive heart failure—the first drug that would be approved for a specific racial group. Other studies have shown similar benefit.[3–5]
- Another analysis suggests a benefit of ISDN/hydralazine in long-term clinical outcomes for a diverse population of patients.[6]

- There is a notable movement within social medicine that recommends the practice of race-conscious medicine over race-based medicine. Instead of providing care based on a supposed biological difference due to race, the recommendation is to provide care on the basis of clinical response to medications and comorbidities, to consider the way structural racism may affect your patients, and to promote resources to reduce racial stress and trauma.[3]
- The 2013 American College of Cardiology Foundation/American Heart Association Task Force guidelines state that a combination of hydralazine and isosorbide dinitrate is recommended "for African Americans with [heart failure with reduced ejection fraction] who remain symptomatic despite concomitant use of Angiotensin-converting enzyme (ACE) inhibitors, beta blockers, and aldosterone antagonists. Whether this benefit is evident in non–African Americans with heart failure with reduced ejection fraction (HFrEF) remains to be investigated."[7]

Summary and Implications: The A-HeFT trial showed that isosorbide dinitrate/hydralazine, when added to standard heart failure therapy, improves outcomes in African Americans with New York Heart Association class III or IV heart failure and a reduced ejection fraction. A-HeFT is also significant because it focused on African American patients, who historically have been underrepresented in medical research.

CLINICAL CASE: TREATMENT OF ADVANCED HEART FAILURE

Case History
A 60-year-old male presenting to the emergency room with dyspnea and lower extremity swelling is diagnosed with class III NYHA congestive heart failure. Near the end of his hospital stay, and after a course of diuretics, the patient will need to be discharged on the appropriate medication. Based on the discussion above, what would be appropriate management for the patient?

Suggested Answer
A-HeFT provided statistically significant data revealing survival benefits in self-identified Blacks with advanced heart failure with the addition of ISDN/hydralazine to standard therapy. According to A-HeFT, this patient

meets criteria for treatment with ISDN/hydralazine combination therapy if he self-identifies as Black. Utilizing this therapy will improve the patient's quality of life and survival rate while decreasing hospitalization. However, if this patient does not self-identify as Black, off-label use of BiDil could be considered depending on his clinical response to other standard therapies and limited evidence that BiDil may also be useful in non-Black patients.

References

1. Taylor AL, Ziesche S, Yancy C, et al. Combination of isosorbide dinitrate and hydralazine in blacks with heart failure. *N Engl J Med*. 2004;351(20):2049–2057.
2. Brody H, Hunt L. BiDil: Assessing a race based pharmaceutical. *Ann Fam Med*. 2006;4(6):556–560.
3. Cerdeña JP, Plaisime MV, Tsai J. From race-based to race-conscious medicine: how anti-racist uprisings call us to act. *Lancet*. 2020;396(10257):1125–1128. doi: 10.1016/S0140-6736(20)32076-6
4. Cohn JN, Johnson G, Ziesche S, et al. A comparison of enalapril with hydralazine–isosorbide dinitrate in the treatment of chronic congestive heart failure. *N Engl J Med*. 1991;325(5):303–310.
5. Ellison GT, Kaufman JS, Head RF, Martin PA, Kahn JD. Flaws in the U.S. Food and Drug Administration's rationale for supporting the development and approval of BiDil as a treatment for heart failure only in black patients. *J Law Med Ethics*. 2008;36(3):449–457. doi: 10.1111/j.1748-720X.2008.290.x
6. Mullens W, Abrahams Z, Francis GS, et al. Usefulness of isosorbide dinitrate and hydralazine as add-on therapy in patients discharged for advanced decompensated heart failure. *Am J Cardiol*. 2009;103(8):1113–1119.
7. Yancy CW, Jessup M, Bozkurt B, Butler J, Casey DE Jr, Drazner MH, Fonarow GC, Geraci SA, Horwich T, Januzzi JL, Johnson MR, Kasper EK, Levy WC, Masoudi FA, McBride PE, McMurray JJ, Mitchell JE, Peterson PN, Riegel B, Sam F, Stevenson LW, Tang WH, Tsai EJ, Wilkoff BL; American College of Cardiology Foundation; American Heart Association Task Force on Practice Guidelines. 2013 ACCF/AHA guideline for the management of heart failure: a report of the American College of Cardiology Foundation/American Heart Association Task Force on Practice Guidelines. *J Am Coll Cardiol*. 2013 Oct 15;62(16):e147–239. doi:10.1016/j.jacc.2013.05.019. Epub 2013 Jun 5. PMID: 23747642.

17

How Do Locals Feel about Expats in Global Health?

JACK FUKUSHIMA AND ARNOLD JUMBE

> Malawian faculty and trainees appreciated the approachability, perspectives, and contribution to education that expatriates have provided, though at times some have been perceived as aggressive, unable to relate to patients and trainees, deficient at adapting to the setting, and self-serving.
>
> —PAREKH ET AL.[1]

Research Question: What are the University of Malawi College of Medicine physicians' and trainees' impressions of expatriate physicians?

Funding: Natasha Parekh was supported by the Health Resources and Services Administration National Research Service Award T32 for Primary Medical Care Research.

Year Study Began: 2014

Year Study Published: 2016

Study Location: University of Malawi College of Medicine, Blantyre, Malawi Who Was Studied: 4th year medical students with clinical experience, interns, registrars, and faculty at the University of Malawi College of Medicine.

Who Was Excluded: The authors of the study did not use exclusion criteria in their sampling.

How Many Subjects: 46

Study Overview: Figure 17.1 provides an overview of the study design. This study was qualitative and used in-depth, semi-structured interviews which were then read, and a codebook was created based on a portion of the interviews. The rest were then read and coded utilizing that codebook. Codes were then reviewed to determine major themes, and representative quotations were chosen.

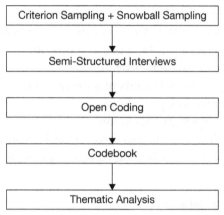

Figure 17.1. Overview of the study design.

Study Intervention: Data were collected through semi-structured interviews.

Follow-Up: This was a single cross-sectional study without follow-up.

Endpoints: Qualitative outcomes, as described below.

RESULTS

Perceived benefits of expatriate physicians in Malawi:
- Positive personality characteristics
  - Expatriate physicians were described as "helpful," "enthusiastic," "hardworking," "motivational," "inspiring."
- Broadened perspectives
  - Expatriate physicians provide diverse perspectives and clinical experiences.
- Reduced feelings of isolation
  - Expatriate physicians allow for Malawian staff to feel connected to "the broader medical community."

- Provision of clinical care
  - Expatriate physicians lessen the burden of clinical care and will sometimes use their personal resources to help patients.

Perceived challenges of expatriate physicians in Malawi:

- Lack of understanding related to culture
- Poor adaptation to low-resourced settings
  - Expatriate physicians sometimes recommend tests and procedures that are unavailable due to resource constraints.
- Communication issues with patients
  - Expatriate physicians' inability to speak the local language limits their ability to engage with patients.
- Self-serving or exploitative intentions
  - Expatriate physicians may put their personal research or clinical ambitions over the needs of the community or local staff.

Criticisms and Limitations:

- The study was conducted at only one institution and thus has limited applicability to other settings.
- The research process was conducted largely by expatriates and the pool of interviewed clinicians is small, potentially leading to selection bias and lack of anonymity among respondents.
- While the authors define "expat," they do not do the same for "locals," an equally nebulous category.

Other Relevant Studies and Information:

- There is a wealth of literature about the ethical considerations of short-term, global health training programs. They point to similar challenges as this study, such as: expatriate trainees having an inflated sense of expertise,[2] unrealistic expectations of expatriates,[2] damaging judgment of local beliefs and traditions on the part of expatriates,[6] etc.
- Other studies and commentaries also make similar recommendations for proactively managing ethical challenges such as: providing trainees with in-depth preparation,[2-4] emphasizing humility and solidarity as core values in these programs,[6] centering reciprocity,[4] and incorporating ethics training as core curriculum in medical school.[7]

• Studies from the social sciences have shown how analyses of value
  structures that have arisen from colonial relationships are necessary
  in order to understand interpersonal relationships and beliefs in the
  context of Global North to Global South programs.[5]

Summary and Implications: This study explores the reflections of physicians
and trainees in Malawi on their expatriate counterparts. They find a number of
impressions, both positive and challenging, that have implications for how to
structure expatriate physician staffing. Through their findings, the authors pro-
pose potential changes to programs that employ the use of expatriate physicians.
They suggest that there be greater communication from the host institution
about expectations; that programs should be designed to foster capacity-building
and sustainability; and that expatriates should prepare themselves before arriving
in the host country by learning a little bit of the language and the history of the
region.

CASE STUDY: A START AT DECOLONIZING GLOBAL HEALTH

Case Overview

As the expatriate coordinator of a medical exchange program in Blantyre,
Malawi, you receive reports from local staff that one of the expatriate physicians
is presenting challenges. They allegedly become frustrated easily when they are
unable to communicate with patients and are quick to reprimand Malawian
staff when they push back against decisions they feel are not appropriate for
their context. When you approach the physician, they claim they are only
trying to provide the best clinical care. What decisions would you make to address this dynamic and prevent future ones from developing?

Suggested Answer

According to the study, such difficulties arise from, among other things, lack
of preparation and clear expectations among all stakeholders. One way to
address the immediate dynamic is to open a dialogue with the expat physician and focus on how they can best provide for the community through
training of local physicians and being open to how lack of resources and other
considerations change medical culture and limit medical care. The physician
might also want to engage in learning the local language to ease some of their
clinical encounters.

This study also points to several programmatic designs that could prevent such interpersonal challenges. As coordinator and an expatriate, you could engage in dialogue with local partners to assure mutual benefit in the outcomes of the exchange program. One way to do this is to explicitly outline the expectations and roles of expatriates and check these against the priorities and needs of local partners.

References

1. Parekh N, Sawatsky AP, Mbata I, Muula AS, Bui T. Malawian impressions of expatriate physicians: A qualitative study. *Malawi Med J.* 2016 Jun;28(2):43–47. doi: 10.4314/mmj.v28i2.3. PMID: 27895827; PMCID: PMC5117098.
2. Crump JA, Sugarman J. Ethical considerations for short-term experiences by trainees in global health. *JAMA.* 2008;300(12):1456–1458. doi: 10.1001/jama.300.12.1456
3. Elit L, Hunt M, Redwood-Campbell L, Ranford J, Adelson N, Schwartz L. Ethical issues encountered by medical students during international health electives. *Med Educ.* 2011;45(7):704–711. doi: 10.1111/j.1365-2923.2011.03936.x
4. Miranda JJ, Garcia PJ, Lescano AG, Gotuzzo E, Garcia HH. Global health training: One way street? *Am J Trop Med Hyg.* 2011;84(3):506; author reply 507. doi: 10.4269/ajtmh.2011.10-0694a
5. Stacy Leigh Pigg; Unintended Consequences: The Ideological Impact of Development in Nepal. *Comparative Studies of South Asia, Africa and the Middle East.* 1993;13(1_and_2):45–58. doi: https://doi.org/10.1215/07323867-13-1_and_2-45
6. Pinto AD, Upshur REG. Global health ethics for students. *Dev World Bioeth.* 2009;9(1):1–10. doi: 10.1111/j.1471-8847.2007.00209.x
7. Shah S, Wu T. The medical student global health experience: professionalism and ethical implications. *J Med Ethics.* 2008;34(5):375–378. doi: 10.1136/jme.2006.019265

18

Azithromycin to Reduce Childhood Mortality in Sub-Saharan Africa

The MORDOR Trial

FRANCES UE

Any policy that recommends mass distribution of oral azithromycin to address childhood mortality would need to consider not only cost but also the risk of side effects, especially the potential for the induction or amplification of antibiotic resistance.

—THE MORDOR (MACROLIDES ORAUX POUR RÉDUIRE LES DÉCÈS AVEC UN OEIL SUR LA RÉSISTANCE) INVESTIGATORS[1]

Research Question: Does twice-yearly mass distributions of oral azithromycin reduce mortality in children 1 to 59 months of age?

Who Funded the Study: Bill and Melinda Gates Foundation

Year Study Began: 2014

Year Study Published: 2018

Study Locations: Malawi (district of Mangochi), Niger (districts of Boboye and Loga), and Tanzania (districts of Kilosa and Gairo)

Who Was Studied: Children 1 to 59 months of age who weighed at least 3800 grams within communities who met the following criteria:

1. The community's location in a target district;
2. The community leader consents to participation in the trial (this does not obviate the need for individual consent, but without overall leadership consent, the community as a whole cannot be part of the trial);
3. Eligible communities have an estimated population of between 200 to 2000 people; and
4. The community is not in an urban area.

Who Was Excluded: Children who had previously received azithromycin.

How Many Patients: 190 328 children

Study Overview: See Figure 18.1.

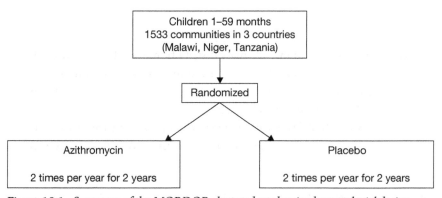

Figure 18.1. Summary of the MORDOR clustered randomized control trial design.

Study Intervention: Children in the azithromycin group received oral azithromycin (at least 20 milligrams per kilogram of body weight), 2 times per year for 2 years. Children in the placebo group received oral placebo during the same time intervals. Children who were known to be allergic to macrolides were not given azithromycin or placebo.

Follow-Up: 2 years

Endpoints:
Primary outcome: all-cause mortality at aggregate, community, country-level.
Secondary outcomes: Subgroup analyses of all-cause mortality by age group and intracensal period, and causes of death based on verbal autopsy.

RESULTS

- Overall all-cause mortality: 14.6 deaths per 1000 person-years in communities that received azithromycin (9.1 in Malawi, 22.5 in Niger, and 5.4 in Tanzania) and 16.5 deaths per 1000 person-years in communities that received placebo (9.6 in Malawi, 27.5 in Niger, and 5.5 in Tanzania).
- Community-level, intention-to-treat analysis showed that overall in all 4 intracensal periods, mortality was 13.5% lower overall (95% confidence interval (CI), 6.7–19.8) in the azithromycin group than in the placebo group (p <0.001).
- Analysis by country showed that mortality rates were lower in the azithromycin group than in the placebo group in all countries, but only with statistical significance in Niger and the greatest risk reduction of 18.1% (95% CI, 10.0–25.5; p <0.001) contributing to the large heterogeneity in the overall study population.
- Analysis by age group showed that children in the youngest age group (1–5 months of age) had the highest overall mortality and largest observed difference in mortality with azithromycin as compared with placebo (24.9% lower with azithromycin; 95% CI, 10.6–37.0; p = 0.001).
- Causes of death were analyzed by a random sample of 250 verbal autopsies from each of the three sites with 41% of deaths due to malaria, 18% due to diarrhea or dysentery, and 12% due to pneumonia.

Criticisms and Limitations:

- The mechanism by which azithromycin reduces mortality is not known. Oral azithromycin has been distributed by the World Health Organization as an effort to eliminate the ocular strains of chlamydia that cause blindness and visual impairment. However, azithromycin also has broad spectrum effects against bacterial pathogens of the lungs and gastrointestinal tract and the reduced mortality observed is likely due to reductions in respiratory infections, diarrhea, and malaria.

Other Relevant Studies and Information:

- The MORDOR Investigators have subsequently published follow-up mortality results[2] and also data on macrolide resistance, which showed increase in erythromycin resistance (12.3%; 95% CI, 5.7–20.0) in the macrolide group compared to the placebo group (2.9%; 95% CI, 0–6.1; p = 0.02).[3]
- Prior results from a cluster-randomized trial[4] and case control trial[5] in an area of Ethiopia in which trachoma is endemic, published in

2009 and 2011, respectively, were the first studies to suggest that mass distribution of azithromycin may reduce childhood mortality.
- The long-term effects of antibiotic resistance are not known, and repeated mass distribution of azithromycin has been shown to garner resistant organisms, in particular macrolide resistance in nasopharyngeal *Streptococcus pneumoniae* and rectal *Escherichia coli*. These difficult-to-treat organisms may potentially reverse any mortality gains, especially in resource-limited settings.
- A follow-up analysis by the MORDOR investigators found that at 2 years, targeted mass treatment with oral azithromycin in preschool children in Niger increased rates of macrolide resistance. Specifically, the proportion of macrolide resistance in nasopharyngeal *Streptococcus pneumoniae* at the community level was higher in the azithromycin group (mean 12.3%; 95% CI, 5.7–20.0) than in the placebo group (mean 2.9%, 95% CI, 0–6.1, $p = 0.02$).[3]
- Macrolides may also induce corrected QT (QTc) interval prolongation, potentiating the risk for arrhythmias, including torsade de pointes and risk of cardiovascular death[6] with a serious warning issued by the U.S. Food and Drug Administration.[7]

Summary and Implications: In this randomized trial in Malawi, Niger, and Tanzania, mass treatment of children 1–59 months of age with azithromycin twice a year was associated with modest but statistically significant reductions in childhood mortality. The findings should be interpreted with caution, however, due to heterogeneity of the results in different regions and among different age cohorts. In addition, more research is needed on the impact of regular mass antibiotic distribution on antibiotic resistance and rare but serious adverse events.

CLINICAL CASE: RISKS AND BENEFITS OF MASS DISTRIBUTION OF AZITHROMYCIN IN SUB-SAHARAN AFRICA

Case History
Through the Millennium Development Goals, there has been substantial progress in reducing under-5 child mortality by more than half around the world. However, despite these advances, the total number of under-5 deaths

remain at 5.2 million worldwide, with the highest rates in sub-Saharan Africa as of 2019.[8]

You are tasked to develop evidence-based strategies to end preventable deaths of under-5 children by 2030 under the United Nations' Sustainable Development Goals (SDGs). Based on the results of the MORDOR trial, would you recommend mass distribution of azithromycin to achieve these mortality targets?

Suggested Answer

The MORDOR trial showed that overall childhood mortality was 13.5% lower in communities who received mass distribution of azithromycin compared to the placebo group, with the greatest risk reduction in Niger and in the youngest age group of 1 to 5 months. Despite these results, there are several serious limitations, including the concern for antibiotic resistance in these communities and their ecosystem at large, and fatal cardiac arrhythmias. There needs to be long-term data regarding antibiotic resistance prior to implementing a policy of mass azithromycin distribution. Furthermore, considering to use a measure that could cause real harm to these individuals and communities highlights the health and structural inequities that contribute to disproportionate under-5 mortality in sub-Saharan Africa, including chemoprevention and treatment of malaria, clean water and sanitation, nutrition, education, and access to primary care.

References

1. Keenan JD, Bailey RL, West SK, et al. Azithromycin to reduce childhood mortality in sub-Saharan Africa. *N Engl J Med*. 2018;378(17):1583–1592.
2. Keenan JD, Arzika AM, Maliki R, et al. Longer-term assessment of azithromycin for reducing childhood mortality in africa. *N Engl J Med*. 2019;380(23):2207–2214.
3. Doan T, Arzika AM, Hinterwirth A, et al. Macrolide resistance in MORDOR I: A cluster-randomized trial in Niger. *N Engl J Med*. 2019;380(23):2271–2273.
4. Porco TC, Gebre T, Ayele B, et al. Effect of mass distribution of azithromycin for trachoma control on overall mortality in Ethiopian children: A randomized trial. *JAMA*. 2009;302(9):962.
5. Keenan JD, Ayele B, Gebre T, et al. Childhood mortality in a cohort treated with mass azithromycin for trachoma. *Clin Infect Dis*. 2011;52(7):883–888.
6. Ray WA, Murray KT, Hall K, et al. Azithromycin and the risk of cardiovascular death. *N Engl J Med*. 2012; 366(20): 1881–1890.
7. FDA Drug Safety Communication: Azithromycin and the risk of potentially fatal heart rhythms. U.S. Food and Drug Administration website. Updated February 14, 2018. Accessed September 10, 2021. https://www.fda.gov/drugs/drug-safety-and-availabil

ity/fda-drug-safety-communication-azithromycin-zithromax-or-zmax-and-risk-pote
ntially-fatal-heart#:~:text=Safety%20Announcement.%20%5B3-12-2013%5D%20
The%20U.S.%20Food%20and%20Drug,lead%20to%20a%20potentially%20fa
tal%20irregular%20heart%20rhythm
8. Children: Improving survival and well-being. World Health Organization website.
   Updated September 8, 2020. Accessed February 4, 2021. https://www.who.int/
   news-room/fact-sheets/detail/children-reducing-mortality

Infectious Diseases and Neglected Tropical Diseases

In this section, we chose to focus on HIV, TB, malaria, diarrhea, pneumonia, and COVID-19. We selected studies on pre-exposure chemoprophylaxis for HIV, prevention of mother-to-child transmission of HIV through breastfeeding, and optimal timing for initiation of HIV treatment. We explored the life-saving development of oral rehydration solution to treat diarrhea from cholera. Similarly, for TB, we chose studies that highlight the importance of household contact investigation, prevention of TB, and treatment for multi-drug-resistant TB. For malaria, we chose a landmark study on prevention using insecticide-treated bed nets and another examining the importance of artesunate in treatment of malaria. We included the SOLIDARITY trial, as it was one of the most extensive adaptive trials on COVID-19 initiated by the World Health Organization (WHO) and provides a model to follow for future global collaborative effort. Finally, we included a study on the use of steroids in meningitis to demonstrate that the efficacy of similar drug regimens may differ depending on health systems and patient populations.

Infectious Diseases and Neglected Tropical Diseases

19

Prevention of HIV

The Partners PrEP Trial

LENA WONG

Oral TDF and TDF-FTC both protect against HIV-1 infection in heterosexual men and women.[1]

Research Question: Can pre-exposure prophylaxis (PrEP) with oral antiretroviral medicines prevent HIV?

Funding: Bill and Melinda Gates Foundation

Year Study Began: 2008

Year Study Ended: 2011

Year Study Published: 2012

Study Location: 4 sites in Kenya and 5 sites in Uganda

Who Was Studied: HIV heterosexual serodiscordant couples

Who Was Excluded: HIV seronegative partner with abnormal renal function, hepatitis B infection, pregnant or breastfeeding; HIV seropositive partner who was taking ART or met national guidelines to start ART.

How Many Patients: 4758 couples enrolled, 4747 followed

Study overview: See Figure 19.1.

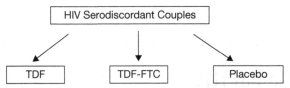

Figure 19.1. Patients were randomized 1:1:1 to take tenofovir (TDF), tenofovir-emtricitabine (TDF-FTC), or placebo daily.

Study Intervention: All participants in both study arms received a comprehensive package of HIV-1 prevention services (HIV-1 testing with counseling), risk-reduction counseling, screening and treatment for sexually transmitted infections, free condoms with training and counseling, and referral for male circumcision and post-exposure prophylaxis according to national policies. Vaccination against hepatitis B virus was also offered. Participants were randomized to TDF, TDF-FTC, or placebo groups in 1:1:1 manner. Seronegative patients had monthly visits with counseling +/– testing, and 30 days of medicines were dispensed. Seropositive patients had quarterly visits, cluster of differentiation 4 (CD4) counts every 6 months, with medications started per guidelines at the time. Patients who became pregnant during the study had medications stopped.

Follow up: 24–36 months, 96% retention

Endpoints: Primary outcome: HIV seropositivity in previously seronegative patients.

RESULTS

- 82 total patients developed HIV infection (1.73%).
  - 17 were in the TDF group.
  - 13 were in the TDF-FTC group.
  - 52 were in the placebo group.
- This trial found an overall relative reduction in HIV acquisition of 67% with TDF alone and 75% with TDF/FTC compared with placebo.
- Across all groups, there was decreased sex without condom use in seronegative partners from 27% at enrollment, down to 13% at 12 months and 9% at 24 months.

- There were no significant differences in the frequency of deaths, serious adverse events, or serum creatinine or phosphorus abnormalities across the study groups.
- The primary reason for stopping the study medication was pregnancy (no difference among groups).

Criticisms and Limitations:

- The study protocol was resource-intensive, requiring frequent staff interactions with patients, which may be difficult to replicate in real-world settings.
- Long-term effects of TDF on renal function and bone density will need further evaluation.

Other Relevant Studies and Information:

- The World Health Organization (WHO) recommends the use of daily oral PrEP as a prevention choice for people at "substantial risk" of HIV infection based in part on this study and others. Substantial risk of HIV infection is defined as HIV incidence greater than 3 per 100 person-years in the absence of PrEP.
- The efficacy of tenofovir for use as PrEP to prevent people from acquiring HIV has been shown in a wide variety of settings and populations that are at substantial risk.[2-4] A previous study on utilizing TDF-FTC in Botswana showed the efficacy of PrEP was 62.2% in the modified intention to treat analysis but was limited by low incidence of HIV and low rate of study completion.[3] A recent population-based study in rural Kenya and Uganda published in 2021 showed 74% lower HIV incidence among PrEP initiators.[5]
- For women at substantial risk of acquiring HIV, there is also a dapivirine vaginal ring (DPV-VR) which can be used as another PrEP option if they are unable or unwilling to use oral PrEP. The Ring Study demonstrated an HIV reduction of 35% among women using DPV-VR, and the ASPIRE study showed a 27% reduction in risk.[6,7]
- Of note, there were some trials showing higher rates of pregnancy among oral contraceptive users who took oral PrEP, but when controlling for confounders this relationship was not significant. Women should be encouraged to continue their birth control method of choice.[4]

- Additionally, there is no evidence that PrEP leads to increased high-risk sexual behavior, such as decreased condom use or more sexual partners.[8]
- Recent data showed efficacy of injectable cabotegravir as PrEP and even superiority over TDF/FTC in HIV-uninfected women.[9]

Summary and Implications: Pre-exposure prophylaxis is an effective way to prevent HIV transmission among heterosexual partners. Global health organizations, such as WHO and the Joint United Nations Programme on HIV/AIDS (UNAIDS), support the use of PrEP in at-risk populations.

CLINICAL CASE: PREVENTING HIV IN SERO-DISCORDANT COUPLES

Case History

A 29-year-old male presents with his female partner to establish care at a new primary provider. He is HIV positive, diagnosed 3 years ago, and takes antiretroviral therapy but has been out of his medication for the past few months. The couple has been together for 1 year and she is HIV negative, last tested 2 weeks ago. They are monogamous but occasionally forget to use condoms. She is on oral contraceptives. How would you further counsel this couple regarding HIV?

Suggested Answer

The couple is monogamous but the risks include an unknown viral load in the HIV seropositive patient, lapse in ART therapy, and inconsistent condom use. The seronegative partner has a recent HIV negative test. The seropositive partner should undergo usual HIV care, including testing for viral load and routine screenings, and both should undergo further testing for other sexually transmitted infections, if not yet already done, and evaluation of renal function. They should be counseled on the use of medications—the seropositive partner for ART therapy and to evaluate if the seronegative partner is willing to consider PrEP therapy. They should be counseled on consistent condom use. She would be a candidate for PrEP therapy, and can continue her oral contraceptive pills.

References

1. Baeten JM, Donnell D, Ndase P, et al. Antiretroviral prophylaxis for HIV prevention in heterosexual men and women. *N Engl J Med*. 2012;367(5):399–410. doi: 10.1056/NEJMoa1108524

2. Grant RM, Lama JR, Anderson PL, et al. Preexposure chemoprophylaxis for HIV prevention in men who have sex with men. *N Engl J Med*. 2010;363:2587–2599.

3. Thigpen MC, Kebaabetswe PM, Paxton LA, et al. Antiretroviral preexposure prophylaxis for heterosexual HIV transmission in Botswana. *N Engl J Med*. 2012;367: 423–434.

4. Fonner VA, Dalglish SL, Kennedy CE, et al. Effectiveness and safety of oral HIV preexposure prophylaxis for all populations. *AIDS*. 2016 Jul 31;30(12):1973–1983.

5. Koss CA, Havlir DV, Ayieko J, et al. HIV incidence after pre-exposure prophylaxis initiation among women and men at elevated HIV risk: A population-based study in rural Kenya and Uganda. *PLoS Med*. 2021 Feb 9;18(2):e1003492. doi: 10.1371/journal.pmed.1003492. PMID: 33561143; PMCID: PMC7872279.

6. Baeten JM, Palanee-Phillips T, Brown ER, et al.; MTN-020–ASPIRE Study Team. Use of a vaginal ring containing dapivirine for HIV-1 prevention in women. *N Engl J Med*. 2016 Dec 1;375(22):2121–2132. doi: 10.1056/NEJMoa1506110. Epub 2016 Feb 22. PMID: 26900902; PMCID: PMC4993693.

7. Nel A, van Niekerk N, Kapiga S, et al.; Ring Study Team. Safety and efficacy of a dapivirine vaginal ring for HIV prevention in women. *N Engl J Med*. 2016 Dec 1;375(22):2133–2143. doi: 10.1056/NEJMoa1602046. PMID: 27959766.

8. Guest G, Shattuck D, Johnson L, et al. Changes in sexual risk behavior among participants in a PrEP HIV prevention trial. *Sex Transm Dis*. 2008;35:1002–1008.

9. Delany-Moretlwe S, Hughes JP, Bock P, et al.; HPTN 084 Study Group. Cabotegravir for the prevention of HIV-1 in women: Results from HPTN 084, a phase 3, randomised clinical trial. *Lancet*. 2022 May 7;399(10337):1779–1789. doi: 10.1016/S0140-6736(22)00538-4. Erratum in: *Lancet*. 2022 May 7;399(10337):1778. PMID: 35378077; PMCID: PMC9077443.

20

Reduced Risk of Post-Natal Transmission of HIV with Extended Antiretroviral Prophylactic Regimen

PEPI Trial (Post-Exposure Prophylaxis of Infants)

TRISHA SCHIMEK

This infant-only anti-retroviral prophylaxis is practical and effective in reducing HIV-1 transmission and in improving HIV-1–free survival in settings in which breast-feeding is common.[1]

Research Question: Does providing infants with extended prophylaxis with nevirapine or nevirapine plus zidovudine until 14 weeks reduce the risk of HIV transmission through breast milk?

Funding: Not stated

Year Study Began: April 2004

Year Study Published: 2008

Study Location: Blantyre, Malawi

Who Was Studied: Breastfeeding infants who were HIV negative at birth who were born to women greater than 18 years with HIV-1.

Who Was Excluded: Women with HIV-1 who were not identified until after birth and infants with life-threatening conditions requiring immediate care. Prophylaxis was discontinued if an infant was found to have HIV-1 infection in the first 14 weeks of life, but they were followed in the study.

How many patients: 3016 breastfeeding infants

Study Overview: See Figure 20.1.

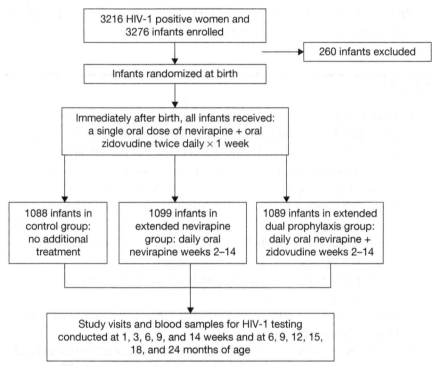

Figure 20.1. Overview of the study design.

Study Intervention: The infants of breastfeeding women infected with HIV-1 were randomly assigned to one of three regimens:

1. Control regimen: Single-dose of nevirapine (2 mg/kg) immediately postpartum plus 1 week of twice daily zidovudine (4 mg/kg). This was the recommended regimen in Malawi for infants born to moms who were not on prophylaxis therapy.
2. Control regimen plus extended prophylaxis with nevirapine for 14 weeks (2 mg/kg daily for week 2 and then 4 mg/kg daily for weeks 3–14).

3. Control regimen plus extended dual prophylaxis of nevirapine plus zidovudine for 14 weeks (4 mg/kg twice daily for weeks 2–5; 4 mg/kg three times daily for weeks 6–8; then 6 mg/kg for three times daily for weeks 9–14).

Follow-Up: Study visits were at 1, 3, 6, 9, 14 weeks and 6, 9, 12, 15, 18, 24 months. Infant blood was collected at each visit to send for HIV-1, CBC (complete blood count), and ALT (alanine aminotransferase test).

Endpoints: Rate of HIV-1 infection confirmed by 2 tests by the age of 9 months among infants who were negative at birth.

RESULTS

- Extended prophylaxis with nevirapine or with nevirapine and zidovudine for the first 14 weeks of life significantly reduced postnatal HIV-1 infection in 9-month-old infants with a protective efficacy of more than 60%.
- The cumulative risk of postnatal infection at 14 weeks was 8.4% in the control group compared to 2.8% in the extended prophylaxis group.
- At 9 months the estimated rate of HIV-1 infection in the control group was 10.6% as compared with 5.2% in the extended-nevirapine group and 6.4% in the extended dual prophylaxis group. The difference between the two extended prophylaxis groups was insignificant.
- The control group had consistently higher rates of HIV-1 infection from 6 weeks through 18 months.
- Extended prophylaxis had higher estimated protective efficacy at 6 weeks, 14 weeks, 6 months, and 9 months.
- Low birth weight was associated with increased risk of HIV infection and death. A decrease in the maternal cluster of differentiation 4 (CD4) cell count was associated with an increased risk of neonatal infection.
- There were 1283 serious adverse events reported among in 887 infants in the study. There were no significant differences between the groups, and the majority of adverse events (87.3%) were not thought to be associated with the study drug. Generally these included respiratory, gastrointestinal, and hematologic events. However, there were more infants with serious adverse events possibly related to the drug in the extended dual prophylaxis group, the most common of which was neutropenia.

Criticisms and Limitations: The 14-week schedule was decided based on the Malawi immunization schedule, thinking the regimen would integrate in a resource-limited setting.

Other Relevant Studies and Information:

- In under-resourced regions, respiratory and gastrointestinal infections are still the leading cause of death in infants. Breastfeeding has been proven to reduce common pediatric illnesses by passing maternal antibodies to the nursing infant, as well as decreasing ingestion of unclean drinking water used in the preparation of formula.
- Without antiviral treatment, the risk of transmission of HIV from infected mothers to their children is approximately 15%–30% during pregnancy and labor, with an additional 10%–20% transmission risk attributed to prolonged breastfeeding.[2]
- Since 2016, World Health Organization (WHO) guidelines have recommended that antiretroviral therapy (ART) be initiated in pregnant and breastfeeding mothers once HIV is identified, as the most effective way to prevent HIV vertical transmission is to reduce maternal viral load. The current WHO HIV[3] guidelines further delineate that all breastfeeding infants receive:
  - Dual prophylaxis with daily nevirapine for 6 weeks
  - Dual prophylaxis with daily azidothymidine (AZT) and NVP for 6 weeks whether breastfeeding or not if they have a higher risk of acquiring HIV (reasons listed below)
  - An additional 6 weeks of either zidovudine and nevirapine or nevirapine alone if they are breastfed and have high risk of acquiring HIV.
- High-risk infants are defined as those born to women:[3]
  - With established HIV infection who have received less than 4 weeks of ART at the time of delivery: or
  - With established HIV infection with viral load >1000 copies/mL in the 4 weeks before delivery, if viral load is available: or
  - With incident HIV infection during pregnancy or breastfeeding: or
  - Identified for the first time during the postpartum period, with or without a negative HIV test prenatally.

Summary and Implications: To avoid transmitting HIV through breastmilk to their baby, some mothers will formula feed instead of breastfeed. In areas where lack of access to clean water is a leading cause of death among infants and children, this alternative may be deadly. This study provides critical information showing that prolonged drug prophylaxis by breastfeeding infants of HIV-positive mothers reduces transmission of HIV from 8.4% to 2.8% in the extended prophylaxis group.

CLINICAL CASE: PREVENTION OF MOTHER TO CHILD TRANSMISSION OF HIV

Case History
A 24-year-old G5P4 woman without any prenatal care presents to a hospital in Malawi when she is in active labor. She has not had access to family planning methods and rarely goes to the clinic except for her child's vaccinations or illness. Her routine perinatal tests reveal that she has HIV with an elevated viral load and CD4 count of 600. Her last child was born 14 months ago and she was told she was HIV negative at the time of her delivery; she breastfed that child up until 9 months. She has heard that she cannot breastfeed because of her HIV, but she does not have money to buy formula or access to clean drinking water and asks what you recommend.

Suggested Answer
This infant is considered at high risk of transmission because the mom was first diagnosed with HIV at time of delivery. She was not taking ART and had an elevated viral load. Since she does not have access to clean drinking water, the WHO recommends breastfeeding to reduce risk of infant morbidity and mortality for all infants regardless of maternal HIV status. The PEPI trial provided data to recommend extended drug prophylaxis after birth for this infant to reduce risk of HIV transmission during breastfeeding. The 2021 WHO guidelines would specifically recommend that this infant receive dual prophylaxis for the first 6 weeks with zidovudine and nevirapine and then an additional 6 weeks of dual prophylaxis or nevirapine alone. Additionally, the mother should continue on ART indefinitely now that she is aware of her HIV diagnosis. Lastly, since it is unknown when she acquired the infection since her last delivery, her youngest child who was breastfeeding and her husband need to be tested for HIV.

References

1. Kumwenda NI, Hoover DR, Mofenson LM, et al. Extended antiretroviral prophylaxis to reduce breast-milk HIV-1 transmission. *N Engl J Med.* 2008 Jul 10;359(2):119–129. doi: 10.1056/NEJMoa0801941. Erratum in: *N Engl J Med.* 2018 Jun 13;null. PMID: 18525035.
2. Volmink J, Marais B. HIV: Mother-to-child transmission. *BMJ Clin Evid.* 2008 Feb 5;2008:0909.
3. WHO Consolidated Guidelines on HIV Prevention, Testing, Treatment, Service Delivery and Monitoring: Recommendations for a Public Health Approach; July 2021. https://www.who.int/publications/i/item/9789240031593

21

When to Start HIV Treatment?
A Global Question

ROBIN GOLDMAN AND GEORGERY CONSTANT

> The benefit of immediate antiretroviral therapy across regions of the
> world indicates that controlling viral replication and improving immune
> function have broad positive effects.
>
> —INSIGHT START TRIAL GROUP[1]

Research Question: Should people living with HIV who have CD4+ counts greater than 500 cells per cubic millimeter (cells/mm^3) and are asymptomatic be started on antiretroviral therapy (ART)?

Funding: National Institute of Allergy and Infectious Diseases and others

Year Study Began: 2009

Year Study Published: 2015

Study Location: 35 countries in the following regions: Africa, Asia, Australia, Europe, Israel, Canada, United States, South America, and Mexico.

Study Participants: HIV-positive patients who were 18 years or older, who had not yet started ART, who had CD4+ counts greater than 500 cells/mm^3 measured twice at least 2 weeks apart within 60 days of enrollment and who were generally healthy.

Who Was Excluded:

1. Patients who had previously been on ART
2. Women who were pregnant or breastfeeding at the time of enrollment
3. Patients who currently or in the past had a clinical AIDS diagnosis
4. Symptoms of HIV progression, severe illness within 6 months prior to enrollment including myocardial infarction, stroke, decompensated liver disease, dialysis, non-AIDS defining cancer, as well as detention or imprisonment.

Number of Participants: 4685

Study Overview: See Figure 21.1.

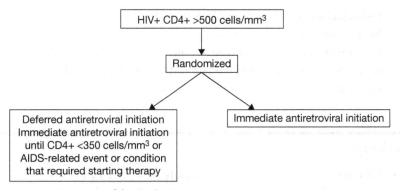

Figure 21.1. Overview of the Study Design.

Study Intervention: The immediate antiretroviral initiation group was started on ART upon enrolling in the study. The deferred antiretroviral initiation group was started on ART when CD4+ counts declined to 350 cells/mm3 or the development of an AIDS-related event or another condition that dictated the use of ART. Regardless of group, when antiretrovirals were initiated, they were a drug combination approved by national guidelines.

Follow-Up: Patients enrolled in the study had follow-up 1 month after enrollment and every 4 months thereafter. The median follow-up time was 2.8 years.

Endpoints: The primary endpoint was a composite of any serious AIDS-related event, including:

1. Death from AIDS or any AIDS-defining event (with the exception of Herpes Simplex virus infection and esophageal candidiasis) and
2. Any serious non-AIDS-related event, including:
    a. Cardiovascular disease (myocardial infarction, stroke, or coronary revascularization)
    b. Death from cardiovascular disease
    c. End-stage renal disease (dialysis or renal transplant) or death from end-stage renal disease
    d. Decompensated liver disease or death from liver disease
    e. Non-AIDS-defining cancer (except basal-cell or squamous-cell skin cancer), death from cancer
    f. Any death not attributable to previously mentioned causes.

Secondary endpoints included:

1. Individual analysis of serious AIDS-related events
2. Serious non-AIDS-related events
3. Death from any cause, life-threatening events not attributable to AIDS, and unscheduled hospitalizations for reasons other than AIDS.

RESULTS

- Characteristics between the immediate (n = 2326) and deferred initiation (n = 2359) groups were similar. Of note, both groups were only 27% women. In the immediate initiation group, patients were on ART for 94% of the follow-up time, compared to 28% of the follow-up time in the deferred initiation group. The percentage of patients with viral suppression after the initiation of ART was similar between groups.
- Results were analyzed based on intention to treat. In both groups the most common events in the composite primary endpoint were cardiovascular disease, non-AIDS-defining cancer, and tuberculosis. The composite primary endpoint occurred in 42 patients in the immediate initiation group and 96 in the deferred initiation group, a hazard ratio of 0.43 for immediate compared to the deferred initiation group (see Table 21.1 for an overview of outcomes).
- Side effects from antiretroviral therapy were low.

Table 21.1

	Immediate Initiation Group n (%)	Deferred Initiation Group n (%)	Hazard Ratio (95% CI)	*p* Value
Composite primary endpoint	42 (1.8%)	96 (4.1%)	0.43 (0.30–0.62)	<0.001
Serious AIDS-related event	14 (0.6%)	50 (2.1%)	0.28 (0.15–0.50)	<0.001
Serious non-AIDS-related event	29 (1.2%)	47 (2.0%)	0.61 (0.38–0.97)	0.04
Death, any cause	12 (0.5%)	21 (0.9%)	0.58 (0.28–1.17)	0.13

Criticism and Limitations:

- While the difference between the early and deferred treatment groups were significant for the composite primary endpoint and some of the individual primary and secondary endpoints, the differences were not significant for all of the individual endpoints in this study. Therefore individual providers will need to take this into account, along with other risk factors, as they counsel patients on the benefits of early initiation of treatment.
- One limitation of the study is that the statistical power for primary events that were attributable to serious non-AIDS-related conditions was lower than expected due to a low number of events during the study period, which means that benefits may not have been precisely quantified.
- The study group was relatively young and the follow-up time of approximately 3 years was relatively short for a chronic disease and lifelong medications. The challenges for patients to adhere to lifelong therapy and the side effects of lifelong ART will need further study. Finally, the coordination of supply chains and cost of starting ART on all persons living with HIV at the international, national, and local levels are not discussed in this article.

Other Relevant Studies and Information:

- The TEMPRANO trial compared an immediate initiation of ART vs. deferred initiation in the Côte d'Ivoire in 849 people. Those started on immediate initiation were significantly less likely to develop an event compared with those who were assigned to deferred therapy (HR 0.56, 95% CI 0.33–0.94).[2]

- In 2015, the World Health Organization announced that it had revised its guidelines to state that everyone diagnosed with HIV should be started on ART, regardless of CD4+ count.[3]

Summary and Implications: Patients with HIV started on ART immediately had health benefits regardless of CD4+ count for both serious AIDS-related and serious non-AIDS-related health conditions. Based on this and other research, major international guidelines now recommend the initiation of ART in all those diagnosed with HIV.

In order to fully realize the goal of starting all persons with HIV on ART, health systems must work on testing infrastructure, supply chain, and patient trust in the healthcare system. In addition, health systems and clinics will need to support, or accompany, patients with lifelong appointments, screening, and treatment.

CLINICAL CASE: INITIATING HIV TREATMENT

Case History
A 29-year-old woman presents to a clinic at a hospital in rural Haiti for a health screening for a new job. As part of her checkup, you order a screening rapid HIV test. The HIV tests returns positive. You order a CD4+ count with her other bloodwork. Based on the START trial, what should you do next?

Suggested Answer
You spend time with the patient discussing her diagnosis. Based on the START trial, you recommend starting treatment immediately and explain this will mean lifelong daily medications even though she is feeling well without symptoms. Based on the START trial, you explain to her that it will lead to improved health over the long term with a decreased risk of HIV-related and non-HIV-related serious health conditions. In addition, you state that this therapy will decrease her risk of infecting others. As her healthcare provider, you must create a partnership that begins at the time of diagnosis and continues through the long duration of her treatment. You also discuss her sexual contacts and recommend they get tested.

Her initial CD4+ count prior to treatment returns at 689 cells/mm³. She continues to take her medications and follow up with you. Six months later, she is still asymptomatic with an increase in her CD4+ count to 748 cells/mm³ and an undetectable HIV viral load. She reports that she has had no health issues since the time of diagnosis.

References

1. INSIGHT START Study Group, Lundgren JD, Babiker AG, et al. Initiation of antiretroviral therapy in early asymptomatic HIV infection. *N Engl J Med*. 2015;373(9):795–807. doi: 10.1056/NEJMoa1506816
2. TEMPRANO ANRS 12136 Study Group, Danel C, Moh R, et al. A trial of early antiretrovirals and isoniazid preventive therapy in Africa. *N Engl J Med*. 2015;373(9):808–822. doi: 10.1056/NEJMoa1507198
3. World Health Organization. *Guideline on When to Start Antiretroviral Therapy and on Pre-exposure Prophylaxis for HIV*; September 2015.

22

Safety and Efficacy of Sulfamethoxazole/ Trimethoprim Chemoprophylaxis for *Pneumocystis carinii* Pneumonia in AIDS

LINDA SHIPTON

The findings of this study demonstrate that sulfamethoxazole and tri-methoprim therapy is effective in preventing P carinii pneumonia in patients with AIDS-associated Kaposi's sarcoma.[1]

Research Question: Is taking sulfamethoxazole and trimethoprim for a prolonged period tolerable and safe, and is it effective in preventing *Pneumocystis carinii* pneumonia in patients with AIDS?

Funding: Not specifically stated

Year Study Began: January 1984

Year Study Published: February 1988

Study Location: Not specifically stated, but patients were predominantly US citizens

Who Was Studied: Patients with a new diagnosis of biopsy-proven Kaposi's sarcoma associated with AIDS were included.

Who Was Excluded: Patients with prior or active opportunistic infections or a sulfonamide allergy were excluded. Patients who had received any prior antiretroviral therapy or chemoprophylactic therapy against *Pneumocystis carinii* were excluded.

How Many Patients: 60

Study Overview: See Figure 22.1

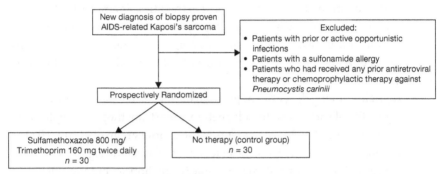

Figure 22.1. Overview of the study design.

Study Intervention: Patients with biopsy-proven Kaposi's sarcoma associated with AIDS were prospectively randomized to receive sulfamethoxazole (800 mg) and trimethoprim (160 mg) twice daily versus no treatment (control group). All patients receiving sulfamethoxazole and trimethoprim received adjunctive leucovorin to combat the anti-folate and bone-marrow-suppressing effects of sulfamethoxazole and trimethoprim. Kaposi's sarcoma was treated per standard of care, and treatment regimens were similar in both groups. Given the year the study was performed, no patient received antiretroviral therapy.

Follow-Up: 24 months

Endpoints:
- Development of a new opportunistic infection, in particular *Pneumocystis carinii* pneumonia
- Length of survival
- Adverse reactions to sulfamethoxazole and trimethoprim

RESULTS

- No patient developed *Pneumocystis carinii* while taking sulfamethoxazole/ trimethoprim prophylaxis compared to 53% in the control group during the course of the study. Within the control group, development of *pneumocystis carinii* was associated with a CD4 count <200 /mm^3, a more advanced stage of Kaposi's sarcoma, and Kaposi's sarcoma subtype B.

- Adverse reactions to sulfamethoxazole/trimethoprim prophylaxis were common; 50% of patients taking sulfamethoxazole/trimethoprim prophylaxis had some reaction, and 17% required discontinuation of the drug due to an adverse reaction.
- The most common reaction was a mild to moderate, nonprogressive erythroderma on the trunk and upper extremities. Severe rash with mucosal involvement and systemic symptoms was the most common reason for drug discontinuation. After drug discontinuation, *Pneumocystis carinii* developed in 80% (4 of 5 patients) of these patients in the following 4–5 months.
- Mortality among the entire population during the course of the study was high: 60% of patients in the sulfamethoxazole/trimethoprim prophylaxis group compared to 93% of patients in the control group died (p <0.02). Among those who died, the mean length of survival was significantly longer in those taking sulfamethoxazole/trimethoprim prophylaxis compared to the control group (22.9 mo vs. 12.6 mo). Opportunistic infections, including *Pneumocystis carinii* in the control group, were the main cause of death in both groups.

Criticisms and Limitations: This was a small study that only included adult men who were predominantly of US citizenship, white, and with homosexual sex as the risk factor for HIV infection. Findings from such a limited study at the time would have needed further verification to prove generalizability to a broader population.

Other Relevant Studies and Information:

- Multiple other subsequent studies have confirmed the findings of this small study, demonstrating the efficacy of trimethoprim/ sulfamethoxazole in preventing *Pneumocystis carinii* pneumonia in patients with AIDS.
- Further studies have shown that lower doses and less frequent dosing of trimethoprim/sulfamethoxazole are efficacious and more tolerable.
- Compared to other prophylactic regimens, including aerosolized pentamidine, dapsone, and atovaquone, trimethoprim/sulfamethoxazole is associated with the lowest risk of developing *Pneumocystis carinii* pneumonia.

- Trimethoprim/sulfamethoxazole prophylaxis in patients with AIDS has also been associated with a lower risk of other infections, including toxoplasmosis, malaria, and severe bacterial infections including diarrheal illnesses, sinusitis/otitis, and pneumonia.
- Both US and international guidelines recommend trimethoprim/sulfamethoxazole as a first-line regimen for prevention of *Pneumocystis carinii* pneumonia in people living with HIV and CD4 count <200.

Summary and Implications: This study, which was performed before antiretroviral therapy was available, was a sentinel study demonstrating that patients with AIDS who took sulfamethoxazole and trimethoprim continuous prophylaxis had a significantly lower risk—approaching zero—of developing *Pneumocystis carinii* pneumonia and an improved survival compared to no therapy. While adverse reactions to the treatment were common, it was tolerated in the majority.

CLINICAL CASE: PREVENTION OF OPPORTUNISTIC INFECTIONS IN PATIENTS WITH HIV

Case History
A 42-year-old male presents to your care with weight loss and fatigue. On review you note that he has had multiple sexually transmitted diseases in the past. HIV testing is done and returns positive with a low CD4 cell count of $73/mm^3$. Other than the weight loss and fatigue, he feels well. There is no clinical evidence of a current opportunistic infection. How do you counsel this patient about the risks and benefits of starting trimethoprim/sulfamethoxazole preventive therapy?

Suggested Answer
While this patient currently has minimal symptoms, the low CD4 count puts him at a significant risk of developing opportunistic infections, most notably *Pneumocystis carinii* pneumonia. In fact, according to this study, without any therapy (antiretroviral or trimethoprim/sulfamethoxazole preventive therapy), he has about a 53% chance of developing *Pneumocystis carinii* pneumonia and a 93% chance of dying over the next several years. Prior to or at the same time as discussing initiation of antiretroviral therapy, you should counsel him about the benefits as well as potential toxicities of starting trimethoprim/sulfamethoxazole for prevention of *Pneumocystis carinii* pneumonia.

Trimethoprim/sulfamethoxazole preventive therapy is highly efficacious in preventing *Pneumocystis carinii* pneumonia. However, side effects, most commonly rash, may occur and can rarely be serious. He should be counseled to call for any concern of a rash and to stop the medication right away if he develops systemic symptoms and/or mucosal involvement.

References

1. Fischl MA, Dickinson GM, La Voie L. Safety and efficacy of sulfamethoxazole and trimethoprim chemoprophylaxis for Pneumocystis carinii pneumonia in AIDS. *JAMA.* 1988;259(8):1185–1189. doi:10.1001/jama.259.8.1185
2. Stansell JD, Osmond DH, Charlebois E, et al. Predictors of *Pneumocystis carinii* pneumonia in HIV-infected persons. Pulmonary Complications of HIV Infection Study Group. *Am J Respir Crit Care Med.* 1997;155(1):60.
3. Dworkin MS, Williamson J, Jones JL, Kaplan JE. Prophylaxis with trimethoprim-sulfamethoxazole for human immunodeficiency virus-infected patients: Impact on risk for infectious diseases. *Clin Infect Dis.* 2001 Aug 1;33(3):393–398.
4. DiRienzo AG, van Der Horst C, Finkelstein DM, Frame P, Bozzette SA, Tashima KT. Efficacy of trimethoprim-sulfamethoxazole for the prevention of bacterial infections in a randomized prophylaxis trial of patients with advanced HIV infection. *AIDS Res Hum Retroviruses.* 2002 Jan 20;18(2):89–94.
5. Panel on Guidelines for the Prevention and Treatment of Opportunistic Infections in Adults and Adolescents with HIV. Guidelines for the Prevention and Treatment of Opportunistic Infections in Adults and Adolescents with HIV. National Institutes of Health, Centers for Disease Control and Prevention, HIV Medicine Association, and Infectious Diseases Society of America. Available at https://clinicalinfo.hiv.gov/en/guidelines/adult-andadolescent-opportunistic-infection. Accessed April 26, 2018. Pages Y-1 - Y-10

23

Isoniazid for Preventing TB in HIV-Positive People

TIMOTHY S. LAUX

Isoniazid preventive therapy should be recommended to all patients receiving antiretroviral therapy in moderate or high [tuberculosis] incidence areas. . . .[1]

Research Question(s): In patients with HIV-1 infection who are starting or continuing antiretroviral therapy (ART) and who do not have active tuberculosis (TB), how effective is 12 months of isoniazid (INH) preventive therapy (IPT) in preventing incident TB disease?

Funding: Multiple (no apparent role for funders)

Year Study Began: 2007

Year Study Published: 2014

Study Location: Ubuntu ART clinic in Cape Town, South Africa

Who Was Studied: Adults with HIV-1 infection on ART

Who Was Excluded:

- <18 years old
- Active TB

- Present or previous latent TB treatment
- Present treatment with antibiotics active against TB
- Issues related to INH (allergy, transaminitis, or neuropathy)
- Pregnancy or ≤6 weeks postpartum

How Many Patients: 1329

Study Overview: See Table 23.1.

Table 23.1 STUDY PROFILE[1]

Recruitment/ Enrollment	Randomization	Excluded	Modified Intention to Treat Analyses
2138 patients assessed	1369 randomized (64.0%), 680 to IPT arm and 689 to placebo arm	40 (2.9%), 18 from IPT arm and 22 from placebo arm (39/40 due to active TB)	1329 analyzed, 662 in IPT arm, 667 in placebo arm; 71 (11%) lost to follow-up in each arm

Study Intervention: Isoniazid (200 or 300 mg PO daily based on weight) or placebo (1:1 ratio, stratified based on ART start) for 12 months.

Follow-Up: Median of 2.5 years per person

Endpoints:
  Primary outcome: Time to development of incident TB, subdivided into definite, probably and possible TB.
  Secondary outcomes: All-cause mortality, adverse drug events/drug discontinuation, durability of treatment effect.

RESULTS

- IPT with ART for HIV-1 positive individuals provided protection against incident TB with a number needed to treat (NNT) of 25. The two combined together likely provide more benefit than either alone (see Table 23.2).
- At enrollment, patients were screened for active (sputum culture) or latent TB (tuberculin skin test [TST] or interferon gamma release assay). Contrary to prior studies,[2,3] this study showed lower hazard ratios for latent TB negative individuals.

- IPT led to no all-cause mortality benefit.
- The number needed to harm (NNH) for stopping was 100.

Table 23.2 SELECTED RESULTS[1]

Outcome	INH		Placebo		Effect
	Events/ person-years	Rate/100 person-years	Events/ person-years	Rate/100 person-years	Unadjusted Hazard Ratio
Incident TB	37/1629.3	2.3	58/1597.2	3.6	0.63 (0.41–0.94)
All-cause mortality	67/1786.3	0.9	21/1792.8	1.2	0.72 (0.34–1.34)
	Events/n	Risk	Events/n	Risk	Unadjusted Relative Risk
Drug discontinuation	102/662	15.4%	94/667	14.1%	1.1 (0.84–1.42)

Criticisms and Limitations:

- Single-center study and thus the findings may not be broadly generalizable
- Among incident TB cases, the majority were classified as "probably/ possible." This raises some concerns about misdiagnosis, especially in settings where TB can be a diagnosis of exclusion due to its myriad presentations and high prevalence.

Other Relevant Studies and Information:

- ART (without INH)[4] and INH (without ART)[2] prevents development of incident TB in HIV-positive individuals.
- In a study from Botswana,[3] 36 months of IPT were more effective for preventing incident TB in HIV-positive individuals than just 6 months of IPT. Unlike this study, the benefit of IPT was predominantly among those with positive TST.
- A 2016 multi-country, open-label, randomized controlled trial was performed that compared IPT to empirical active TB treatment in those with advanced HIV (CD4 <50 cells/microL) starting ART.[5] The primary endpoint was mortality at 24 weeks. Empiric TB treatment did not reduce mortality compared with IPT.

Summary and Implications: In moderate- or high-burden TB settings, HIV-1 positive individuals on ART should receive 12 months of weight based IPT (with pyridoxine) for prevention of incident TB, regardless of the results of latent TB testing, unless contraindicated (e.g.. due to underlying liver disease or the development of INH-induced hepatotoxicity or neurotoxicity). This recommendation comes with the underlying assumptions: (1) active TB infection can be ruled out, and (2) outpatient follow-up can be performed regularly to monitor for adverse drug events (ADEs).

CLINICAL CASE: PREVENTION OF TB IN HIV POSITIVE PATIENTS

Case History

A 29-year-old woman with no past medical history presents with oral thrush and weight loss (from 60 to 45 kg). Testing reveals HIV-1 antibodies. Her viral load is elevated and her CD4 count 42 cells/microL (18%).

She reports a rare, chronic cough, which she attributes to allergies. A chest x-ray is clear with a negative sputum acid fast bacilli (AFB) X 3 and a negative cartridge-based nucleic acid amplification test (CBNAAT). Sputum culture is pending. She is not pregnant. Her labs show normal transaminase levels. She lives in a community with a high burden of TB disease. She has never been treated for latent or active TB.

In addition to starting the patient on ART (and appropriate opportunistic infection prophylaxis), what can you do to prevent her from developing incident TB?

Suggested Answer

It is entirely possible that this young woman already has active TB infection though it remains subclinical and would be classified as sputum negative. It is very important that her sputum culture be followed up. In the meantime, she should be started on IPT which should either be (1) continued when sputum culture is negative for 12 months or (2) discontinued and transitioned to active TB treatment with medications to which her TB is susceptible if the sputum culture returns as positive.

Initially, she should receive INH 200 mg PO daily and pyridoxine 25 mg PO daily. If her weight increases to ≥50 kg, she should be transitioned to INH 300 mg PO daily.

Finally, she will need ongoing, regular follow-up to monitor her response to ART, any adverse drug effects of INH, and medication adherence.

References

1. Rangaka MX, Wilkinson RJ, Boulle A, et al. Isoniazid plus antiretroviral therapy to prevent tuberculosis: A randomised double-blind, placebo-controlled trial. *Lancet.* 2014;384:682–690.
2. Akolo C, Adetifa I, Shepperd S, Volmink J. Treatment of latent tuberculosis infection in HIV infected persons. *Cochrane Database Syst Rev.* 2010;2010(1):CD000171. Published 2010 Jan 20. doi:10.1002/14651858.CD000171.pub3
3. Samandari T, Agizew TB, Nyirenda S, et al. 6-month versus 36-month isoniazid preventive treatment for tuberculosis in adults with HIV infection in Botswana: A randomised, double-blind, placebo-controlled trial. *Lancet.* 2011;377:1588–1598.
4. Suthar AB, Lawn SD, del Amo J, et al. Antiretroviral therapy for prevention of tuberculosis in adults with HIV: A systematic review and meta-analysis. *PLoS Med.* 2012;9:e1001270.
5. Hosseinipour MC, Bisson GP, Miyahara S, et al. Empirical tuberculosis therapy versus isoniazid in adult outpatients with advanced HIV initiating antiretroviral therapy (REMEMBER): A multicountry open-label randomised controlled trial. *Lancet.* 2016;387:1198–1209.

Impact of Improved Treatment of Sexually Transmitted Diseases on HIV Infection in Rural Tanzania

Randomized Controlled Trial

CASEY SAUTTER, RYAN SHIELDS, AND
SADOSCAR HAKIZIMANA

We conclude that improved STD treatment reduced HIV incidence by
about 40% in this rural population. This is the first randomised trial to
demonstrate an impact of a preventive intervention on HIV incidence in
a general population.

—GROSSKURTH ET AL.[1]

Research Question: What is the impact of an improved sexually transmitted disease (STD) treatment program on HIV incidence?

Funding: The European Communities (DGVIII), with additional funds from the UK Overseas Development Administration, the EC Life Sciences and Technologies for Developing Countries, the Centre for International Migration program and Development, Germany, and the UK Medical Research Council

Year Study Began: 1991

Year Study Published: 1995

Study Location: Mwanza region of Tanzania

Who Was Studied: 6 matched and paired community cohorts from a variety of geographical locations within a 90-minute walking distance from the local health center.

Who Was Excluded: Cohort members who moved, were temporarily absent, died, refused, or were inaccessible at the time of follow-up.

How many participants: 12 537

Study overview: See Figure 24.1

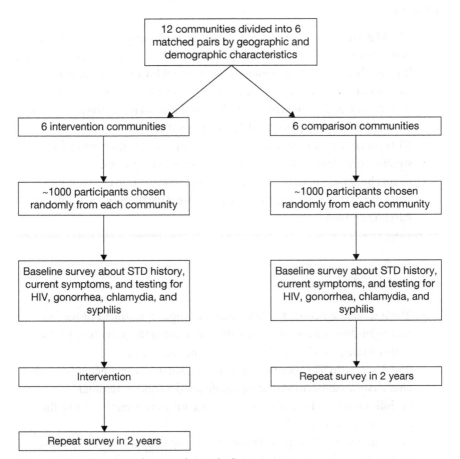

Figure 24.1. Flowchart showing the study design.

Study Intervention: The intervention consisted of establishing a reference STD lab, supplying medications for syndromic STD treatment, a 3-week training for health center professionals on syndromic treatment, periodic health education in included villages, and routine supervisory visits to the health centers.

Follow-up: 2 years

Endpoints:

Primary outcome: Incidence of HIV infection

Secondary outcomes: Prevalence of STDs (gonorrhea, chlamydia, syphilis, presumed symptomatic infection); self-assessed sexual behaviors (number of partners in past year, number of casual partners in past 2 years)

RESULTS

- 12 537 participants were enrolled at baseline from sampled households and 8845 were resurveyed and tested at the 2-year follow-up, a 71% follow-up rate.
- The incidence of HIV seroconversion was 42% lower in intervention communities (48 seroconversions or 1.2% rate vs. 82 seroconversions or 1.9% rate in the intervention and control groups respectively, with an adjusted RR of 0.58 [95% CI 0.42–0.79, $p = 0.007$]).
- STD prevalence at follow-up was lower in the intervention group but not significantly different between the two community groups.
- Sexual behaviors between comparison and intervention communities (lifetime partners, partners in past year, casual partners) were similar at baseline and follow-up.

Criticisms and Limitations:

- The intervention consisted of syndromic empiric treatment instead of pathogen-directed treatment and did not address the potential pitfalls of this strategy, such as multidrug-resistant gonorrhea.
- The decrease in STD prevalence was not statistically significant (though later analyses did demonstrate a significant decrease in serologic syphilis rates)[2] and thus the observed outcomes may not be due to the actual intervention itself.
- This study may not be generalizable to all populations, especially those with a more advanced HIV epidemic with higher prevalence rates.[3]

Other Relevant Studies and Information:

- The Rakai trial performed in Uganda was another community-randomized controlled trial exploring the effect of empiric, periodic mass treatment of STDs on the incidence of HIV-1. After 3 rounds of mass treatment, a mid-trial analysis failed to show any reduction in the incidence of HIV-1 and the trial was stopped early.[4,5] These results seemingly contradicted the results of the trial in Mwanza. However, the Mwanza trial studied the effect of prevention bundles in an area of lower baseline HIV-1 prevalence, whereas the Rakai trial focused on empiric mass treatment in an area with higher baseline prevalence of HIV-1. Thus, the effect of STDs may be blunted in areas, like Rakai, with a higher prevalence of HIV.
- On further analysis of the Rakai trial, the HIV viral load was found to be the main determinant of HIV-1 transmission,[6] suggesting that different prevention approaches may be needed in areas that are in different stages of the HIV epidemic.
- Syndromic management of STDs is promoted by the World Health Organization (WHO), particularly in low-resource settings that lack laboratory capacity and trained personnel. This approach has led to decreased rates of STDs in a variety of settings.[7] However, many studies have also shown the limitations of syndromic treatment;[8] it is also important to continuously reconsider the approach in light of changes such as increasing rates of antibiotic resistant gonorrhea and faster, cheaper etiologic testing.

Summary and Implications: This community-level randomized controlled trial showed that a bundle of population-based interventions aimed at preventing and empirically treating STDs can considerably decrease the incidence of HIV in rural communities by about 40%.

CLINICAL CASE: EMPIRIC TREATMENT FOR SEXUALLY TRANSMITTED INFECTIONS USING A MULTIPRONGED APPROACH

Case History

You are working for the Rwandan Ministry of Health with a focus on reproductive health. A district in the southwest of the country has higher rates of STDs (including HIV) than elsewhere. You are tasked to develop a strategy to help prevent further infections. What would you include in your program development?

Suggested Answer

It is now well known that co-infection with other STDs increases the risk of transmission and susceptibility to HIV, as shown above and in numerous other studies from a variety of settings.[6] This is especially true for ulcerative STDs, including herpes simplex virus, syphilis, and *H ducreyi*.[4,5,9-11] In addition to condom use, harm reduction education, and circumcision, treatment of concurrent STDs can also play a role in HIV prevention, expanding on its importance in reproductive health.

To build a program to reduce rates of STDs, initial testing to establish baseline prevalence and antimicrobial sensitivity patterns is important to distinguish between symptomatically similar STDs. As the methodology of this article makes clear, there needs to be a focus on health systems in order to create sustainable systemic change. Such considerations include: (1) establishing an STD reference clinic and laboratory; (2) training staff in the diagnosis of and syndromic treatment algorithms for STDs; (3) ensuring a regular supply of medications used to treat STDs; (4) regular supervisory visits to provide training, check drug supplies, and review patient records; and (5) intermittent educational outreach to the villages to provide information on STDs.

Expanding from the findings in this study, it would be important to also consider rapid point-of-care testing, testing of asymptomatic patients, HPV vaccine implementation, and expedited partner therapy as possible components in any intervention.

References

1. Grosskurth H, Mosha F, Todd J, Mwijarubi E, Klokke A, Senkoro K, Mayaud P, Changalucha J, Nicoll A, ka-Gina G, Newell J, Mugeye K, Mabey D, Hayes R. Impact of improved treatment of sexually transmitted diseases on HIV infection in rural Tanzania: Randomised controlled trial. *Lancet*. 1995 Aug 26;346(8974):530–536. doi:10.1016/s0140-6736(95)91380-7. PMID: 7658778.

2. Mayaud P, Mosha F, Todd J, Balira R, Mgara J, West B, Rusizoka M, Mwijarubi E, Gabone R, Gavyole A, Grosskurth H, Hayes R, Mabey D. Improved treatment services significantly reduce the prevalence of sexually transmitted diseases in rural Tanzania: Results of a randomized controlled trial. *AIDS*. 1997 Dec;11(15):1873–1880. doi:10.1097/00002030-199715000-00013. PMID: 9412707.

3. Fleming DT, Wasserheit JN. From epidemiological synergy to public health policy and practice: The contribution of other sexually transmitted diseases to sexual transmission of HIV infection. *Sex Transm Infect*. 1999 Feb;75(1):3–17. doi:10.1136/sti.75.1.3. PMID: 10448335; PMCID: PMC1758168.

4. Wawer MJ, Gray RH, Sewankambo NK, et al. A randomised, community-based trial of intense sexually transmitted disease control for AIDS prevention, Rakai, Uganda. *AIDS*. 1998;12:1211–1225.

5. Wawer MJ, Sewankambo N, Serwadda D, et al. Control of sexually transmitted diseases for AIDS prevention in Uganda: A randomised community trial. *Lancet*. 1999;353:525–535.

6. Quinn TC, Wawer MJ, Sewankambo NK, et al. Viral load and heterosexual transmission of human immune deficiency virus type 1. *N Engl J Med*. 2000;342:921–929.

7. World Health Organization. Global health sector strategy on sexually transmitted infections 2016–2021. Towards ending STIs. Report. Geneva: 2016 June. Report No.: WHO/RHR/16.09.

8. Garrett NJ, Osman F, Maharaj B, Naicker N, Gibbs A, Norman E, Samsunder N, Ngobese H, Mitchev N, Singh R, Abdool Karim SS, Kharsany ABM, Mlisana K, Rompalo A, Mindel A. Beyond syndromic management: Opportunities for diagnosis-based treatment of sexually transmitted infections in low- and middle-income countries. *PLoS One*. 2018 Apr 24;13(4):e0196209. doi:10.1371/journal.pone.0196209. PMID: 29689080; PMCID: PMC5918163.

9. Freeman EE, Weiss HA, Glynn JR, Cross PL, Whitworth JA, Hayes RJ. Herpes simplex virus 2 infection increases HIV acquisition in men and women: Systematic review and meta-analysis of longitudinal studies. *AIDS*. 2006 Jan 2;20(1):73–83. doi:10.1097/01.aids.0000198081.09337.a7. PMID: 16327322.

10. Reynolds SJ, Risbud AR, Shepherd ME, Rompalo AM, Ghate MV, Godbole SV, Joshi SN, Divekar AD, Gangakhedkar RR, Bollinger RC, Mehendale SM. High rates of syphilis among STI patients are contributing to the spread of HIV-1 in India. *Sex Transm Infect*. 2006 Apr;82(2):121–126. doi:10.1136/sti.2005.015040. PMID: 16581736; PMCID: PMC2564682.

11. Wawer MJ, Gray RH, Sewankambo NK, Serwadda D, Li X, Laeyendecker O, Kiwanuka N, Kigozi G, Kiddugavu M, Lutalo T, Nalugoda F, Wabwire-Mangen F, Meehan MP, Quinn TC. Rates of HIV-1 transmission per coital act, by stage of HIV-1 infection, in Rakai, Uganda. *J Infect Dis*. 2005 May 1;191(9):1403–1409. doi:10.1086/429411. Epub 2005 Mar 30. PMID: 15809897.

25

A National Program to Introduce Impregnated Bednets to Address Malaria in Gambia

JESSICA C. PARKER

In a country such as The Gambia, where nets were widely used and which has a good primary health care system, it is possible to achieve insecticide-treatment of bednets at a national level with a significant reduction in child mortality; but at a cost which the country cannot afford.[1]

Research Question: Does the implementation of a national program to introduce impregnated bednets into communities reduce morbidity and mortality from malaria in Gambian children age 1–9?

Funding: UNDP/World Bank/WHO Special Programme for Research and Training in Tropical Diseases

Year Study Began: 1992

Year Study Published: 1995

Study Location: 5 distinct, large villages in The Gambia

Who Was Studied: Children age 1 month–9

Who Was Excluded: Gambian children over age 9, and children less than 1 month of age

How Many Patients: 41 102

Study Overview: See Figure 25.1.

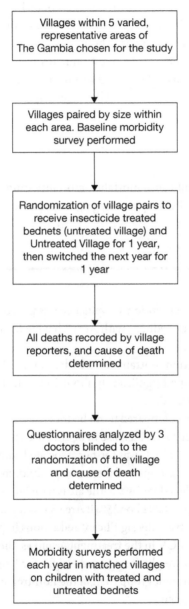

Figure 25.1. Summary of the study's design.

Study Intervention: Five separate geographic areas in The Gambia were chosen to be evaluated, and within each region villages were chosen and matched based on size. Baseline data were collected on pre-intervention use of bednets in addition to baseline childhood morbidity and mortality. After 1 year of surveillance, the villages were randomized to receive treatment for their bednets or no treatment for 1 year, and then the treatment and control villages were switched for 1 year. The deaths of children age 1–9 years were recorded by Medical Record Field Assistants, and questionnaires about the circumstances of the child's death were given to the parents. These questionnaires were then reviewed by three doctors for probable cause of death. Data for thick and thin blood films to look at malaria, mean packed-cell volume (PCV), and splenomegaly were obtained to help determine morbidity.

Follow-Up: One year

Endpoints: Rates of all-cause mortality, mortality from malaria, and morbidity as determined by low PCV, splenomegaly, or evidence of parasitemia on thick and thin blood films

RESULTS

- During the pre-intervention surveillance it was noted that not all areas had uniform use of bednets, with Area 3 having the highest use and Area 5 with the lowest use.
- The pre-intervention mortality for children under 9 was similar across all areas and dropped significantly about 1 month after the impregnated bednets were initiated.
- The use of bednets compared to no bednet use decreases mortality by a rate of 8% for every 10% increase in bednet use ($p = 0.01$).
- The use of treated bednets was further associated with a decrease in all-cause mortality in all age groups and areas except children age 1–2 in Area 5. Mortality was reduced by 38% in the areas with impregnated bednets if Area 5 was excluded ($p = 0.001$) or 25% if Area 5 was included ($p = 0.04$).
- There were no statistically significant reductions in parasitaemia, splenomegaly, or PCV in the treatment group vs. the non-treatment group.
- Mean z-scores for weight-for-age and weight-for-height were statistically higher in the treatment group than in the non-treatment group ($p = 0.008$, $p = 0.001$, respectively).
- This campaign cost approximately US$92 000, 60% of which was attributed to the cost of insecticide, and would need to be repeated yearly.
- Table 25.1 shows a statistically significant 25% decrease in all-cause mortality in the treatment group with impregnated bednets.

Table 25.1 SUMMARY OF THE STUDY'S KEY FINDINGS

All-cause mortality	Child Age 1–2 years	3–4 years	5–9 years	All Ages
RR*	0.95	0.55	0.53	0.75
95% CI	0.71–1.28	0.3–1.01	0.28–0.99	0.57–0.98
p value	0.75	0.05	0.05	0.04

* Rate Ratio (RR) from Multivariate Poisson Model.

Criticisms and Limitations:

- The method of determining cause of death by malaria was subjective, undertaken by questionnaire administered to each child's parent. While the results were evaluated by blinded third parties, there could have been deaths that were inappropriately attributed to malaria or deaths due to malaria that were missed. Additionally, only 79% of the questionnaires were collected, and the methods do not specify what questions were asked in order to determine cause of death by malaria.
- The study populations had poor compliance with bednet implementation, with some areas under investigation only using bednets 56% of the time.
- The national program was designed only to treat the nets of those who already owned a bednet, resulting in a lack of representation of families who either cannot afford the nets or who choose not to purchase nets.

Other Relevant Studies and Information:

- Smaller scale trials and a large controlled trial showed promise that bednet use and especially permethrin-impregnated bednet use could decrease mortality in Gambian children.[3-5] However, it was unclear if these results would be as robust in the context of real-world application. The National Insecticide Impregnated Bednet Programme (NIBP) discussed above was in response to this larger controlled trial in hopes to increase impregnated bednet use in all large villages in The Gambia and to evaluate its impact when implemented as part of a public health program.
- Implementing such programs can be a significant cost burden on the health system. Another trial evaluated the use of a small fee to offset the cost of the program. During the first year of this study, insecticide

was distributed free of charge and 80% of existing nets were treated with insecticide, with a 25% decrease in all-cause mortality. However, the following year a small fee was charged, which resulted in a drop in uptake (only 14%) and no resultant impact on mortality.[6]

• A later study performed in Tanzania used careful marketing research to educate patients on the benefits of insecticide-treated nets and utilized culturally appropriate product promotion with appropriate pricing based on the local population's willingness and ability to pay. This resulted in rapid increase of net ownership (10% to 61%) and treatment of nets, as well as a dramatic decrease of anemia (49% to 26%), as well as parasitemia, and splenomegaly in children under 2 years of age.[2]

Summary and Implications: This study showed that the use of insecticide-treated bednets at a national level will result in a significant reduction in child mortality. However, the cost of insecticide may be prohibitive to perform this intervention on a large scale in low-income nations.

CLINICAL CASE: ARE BEDNETS WORTH THE COST?

Case History

While working in The Gambia, you are approached by the director of the clinic. They indicate to you that death rates in the local population have gone up exponentially, largely due to malaria—especially among children. He has heard about a neighboring village that has been using insecticide-treated bednets with some success, and he asks you if you would recommend that his village try something similar. He indicates to you that based on a lack of government funding, cost is an issue. Are there data to support a childhood mortality benefit when using insecticide-treated bednets?

Suggested Answer

This study and similar earlier studies demonstrate a clear childhood mortality benefit to using insecticide-treated bednets compared with untreated bednets, but both are better than no net at all. This benefit appears to correlate with compliance and is most profound when bednets are reliably used. Unfortunately, these results come with the caveat that it may be a fairly cost-prohibitive strategy.

One way to respond to this clinic director would be to indicate that there is a definite mortality benefit to using insecticide-treated bednets, especially among children under 9. It should be stressed that in addition to lowering mortality rates, data demonstrate a decrease in the rates of parasitemia and splenomegaly, indicating lower parasite burden. It would be prudent to stress that these results improve with higher rates of compliance, so explaining proper dilution and utilization of insecticide is paramount. Additionally, it would be necessary to explain that insecticide is costly, so if the clinic was unable to manage the price, they may need to reach out to global relief organizations for additional assistance and/or perform research to determine the best ways to encourage bednet use and prioritization among families, as well as the ability and willingness of those receiving the treated nets to cost-share.

References

1. D'Alessandro U, Olaleye BO, McGuire W, et al. Mortality and morbidity from malaria in Gambian children after introduction of an impregnated bednet programme. *Lancet.* 1995 Feb 25;345(8948):479–483. doi: 10.1016/s0140-6736(95)90582-0. PMID: 7861874.
2. Abdulla S, Schellenberg JA, Nathan R, et al. Impact on malaria morbidity of a programme supplying insecticide treated nets in children aged under 2 years in Tanzania: community cross sectional study. *BMJ.* 2001;322(7281):270–273. doi: 10.1136/bmj.322.7281.270
3. Alonso PL, Lindsay SW, Armstrong JR, et al. The effect of insecticide-treated bed nets on mortality of Gambian children. *Lancet.* 1991;337(8756):1499–1502. doi:10.1016/0140-6736(91)93194-e
4. Snow RW, Rowan KM, Greenwood BM. A trial of permethrin-treated bed nets in the prevention of malaria in Gambian children. *Trans R Soc Trop Med Hyg.* 1987;81:563–567.
5. Snow RW, Rowan KM, Lindsay SW, Greenwood BM. A trial of bed nets (mosquito nets) as a malaria control strategy in a rural area of The Gambia, West Africa. *Trans R Soc Trop Med Hyg.* 1988;82:212–216.
6. Cham K, Olaleye B, D'Alessandro U, et al. The impact of the introduction of cost recovery on the Gambian National Impregnated Bednet Programme. *Health Policy Plan.* 1997;12:240–247.

26

Artesunate versus Quinine for Severe *Falciparum* Malaria

The South East Asian Quinine Artesunate Malaria Trial (SEAQUAMAT)

ANURIMA BAIDYA

For adults with severe malaria, artesunate should be the treatment of choice. The drug is more effective than quinine, is simple to administer, and is safe.

—THE SEAQUAMAT AUTHORS[1]

Research Question: Should patients diagnosed with severe malaria be managed with parenteral artesunate or parenteral quinine?

Funding: Wellcome Trust

Year Study Began: 2003

Year Study Published: 2005

Study Location: Bangladesh, Myanmar, India, and Indonesia

Who Was Studied: Patients diagnosed with severe malaria as determined by the admitting physician, greater than 2 years of age. In addition, a confirmatory diagnosis of malaria by a positive blood antigen stick test for *Plasmodium falciparum* histidine-rich protein (HRP2) was an eligibility criterion.

Who Was Excluded: Patients with a recorded past history of complete treatment with quinine or an artemisinin derivative for more than 24 hours before admission, or if there was any pertinent history of allergic reaction to one of the artemisinin derivatives or quinine.

How Many Patients: 1461 patients

Study Overview: See Figure 26.1.

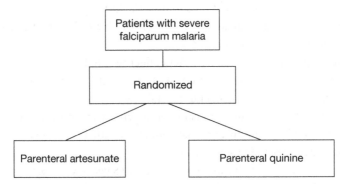

Figure 26.1. Summary of SEAQUAMAT Design.

Study Intervention: Patients randomized to the parenteral artesunate group were administered 2.4 mg/kg body weight on admission, followed by subsequent doses at 12 and 24 hours. This was followed by one daily dosage until the patient tolerated oral medication. Oral artesunate was administered as 2 mg salt per kg per day for a total duration of 7 days and provided a total cumulative dose of 17–18 mg/kg.

Patients randomized to the parenteral quinine group were initiated on a 20 mg/kg loading dose of quinine dihydrochloride infused over 4 hours. Thereafter, the amount was titrated to 10 ml/kg infusion over 2 to 8 hours three times a day until the patient tolerated oral therapy. Oral quinine was administered at a dose of 10 mg/kg every 8 hours over a total duration of 7 days.

Additionally, study patients were administered oral doxycycline at a dose of 100 mg twice a day for seven days once they were capable of oral intake, except in children less than 8 years or pregnant women and at study sites located in Chittagong, Bangladesh, or Orissa, India.

Follow-Up: 2 years

Endpoints:
Primary outcomes: In-hospital mortality due to severe malaria.

Secondary outcomes: new-onset neurological sequelae, the composite outcome of death or neurological sequelae, time to recovery (times to eat, speak, sit, discharge), and rates of severe complications.

RESULTS

- In the artesunate group, 70% of individuals were diagnosed with severe disease compared to 74% in the quinine group.
- Overall mortality was estimated to be 19%. In-hospital mortality in the group receiving artesunate was 15% compared with 22% in the group receiving quinine (see Table 26.1).
- A major proportion of the treatment effect resulted from a reduction in mortality, observed after the first 24–48 hours after entry to the study.
- Significant differences in overall mortality were noted for the participating countries; however, no significant heterogeneity was observed in the treatment effect. The absolute risk reduction with artesunate treatment ranged from 5% to 9% across countries.
- Overall mortality in children younger than 15 years was 8%, but the study did not report any significant difference for the primary outcome of mortality between the two treatment groups in this sub-population.
- There were no significant differences between the two treatment groups for the secondary outcomes looking at times to speak, eat, sit, or be discharged.
- Hypoglycemia was observed predominantly in the quinine group compared with the artesunate group (RR 3.2, 95% CI 1.3–7.8)

Table 26.1 SUMMARY OF KEY FINDINGS OF SAEQUAMAT

Outcome	Parenteral Artesunate	Parenteral Quinine	*p* Value
In-hospital mortality	15%	22%	0.0002
Neurological sequelae	1%	<1%	0.22
The combined outcome of in-hospital mortality or neurological sequelae	16%	23%	0.0007

Criticisms and Limitations:

- First, the trial did not find any significant reduction in mortality between the two groups among children, which warrants further investigation. Prior evidence suggests that younger children have a greater likelihood of presenting with severe malaria, specifically in areas of high transmission.

- Second, the study did not observe any significant difference with regard to secondary outcomes, including neurological sequelae, shock, blackwater fever, convulsions, and mechanical ventilation, between the two study populations. Thus, the underlying causes of deaths predominantly noted in the quinine group remain to be ascertained.
- Third, hypoglycemia observed in 3% of the study participants is probably an underestimation and highlights the need for continuous monitoring in high-risk patients.
- Fourth, the study was conducted in areas of high endemicity but low transmission, which may not apply to sub-Saharan Africa with documented pockets of high malaria transmission.

Other Relevant Studies and Information:

- A meta-analysis of pooled data from 16 randomized control trials reported that a treatment regimen consisting of 3 days of artesunate in conjunction with standard antimalarial treatments could considerably reduce parasitological failure, gametocyte count, and recrudescence.[1]
- Several randomized controlled trials with smaller sample sizes in different geographic locations substantiated the results of this study.[2-5]
- Another landmark trial conducted in 11 centers across 9 African countries among children younger than 15 years concluded that artesunate substantially reduces mortality and morbidity in African children with severe malaria.[6]

Summary and Implications: This multi-center, open-label, randomized trial determined that parenteral artesunate effectively reduces mortality and should become the treatment of choice for severe *P. falciparum* malaria cases in adults. These findings, however, may not be generalizable to the pediatric population.

CLINICAL CASE: ARTESUNATE VS. QUININE IN TREATMENT OF SEVERE MALARIA

Case History

A 56-year-old street food vendor with type 2 diabetes presents with a 5-day history of fever, headache, myalgias, nausea, and anorexia with no significant past medical history of prior malarial or flavivirus infections, chronic illnesses, jaundice, or liver or kidney disorders. On admission, he was found to be febrile

(100.3°F), with a GCS of 15/15, blood pressure of 87/52 mmHg, heart rate 105 beats per minute, and respiratory rate of 36 breaths/minute. Rapid diagnostic test confirms the diagnosis of malaria. Subsequent blood tests confirmed a diagnosis of severe *P. falciparum* malaria based on hyperparasitaemia.

Based on the results of SEAQUAMAT, how should this patient be treated?

Suggested Answer

SEAQUAMAT showed that artesunate effectively reduces mortality due to severe malaria compared to quinine, and the rate of hypoglycemia is lower in the group treated with artesunate. Based on these findings, intravenous artesunate may be the preferred strategy for managing this patient.

The patient presented here is typical of patients included in SEAQUAMAT. Therefore, he can be initiated on 2.4 mg/kg body weight of parenteral artesunate. Careful monitoring of blood glucose concentration is required in this case, as the patient has diabetes and is currently under regular medication.

References

1. Adjuik M, Babiker A, Garner P, et al. Artesunate combinations for treatment of malaria: meta-analysis. *Lancet.* 2004;363(9402):9–17. https://doi.org/10.1016/s0140-6736(03)15162-8
2. Tran TH, Day NP, Nguyen HP, et al. A controlled trial of artemether or quinine in Vietnamese adults with severe falciparum malaria. *New Engl J Med.* 1996;335(2):76–83. https://doi.org/10.1056/NEJM199607113350202
3. Newton PN, Angus BJ, Chierakul W, et al. Randomized comparison of artesunate and quinine in the treatment of severe falciparum malaria. *Clin Infect Dis.* 2003;37(1):7–16.
4. Win K, Than M, Thwe Y. Comparison of combinations of parenteral artemisinin derivatives plus oral mefloquine with intravenous quinine plus oral tetracycline for treating cerebral malaria. *Bull World Health Organ.* 1992;70(6):777–782.
5. Cao XT, Bethell DB, Pham TP, et al. Comparison of artemisinin suppositories, intramuscular artesunate and intravenous quinine for the treatment of severe childhood malaria. *Trans R Soc Trop.* 1997;91(3):335–342. https://doi.org/10.1016/s0035-9203(97)90099-7
6. Dondorp AM, Fanello CI, Hendriksen IC, et al. Artesunate versus quinine in the treatment of severe falciparum malaria in African children (AQUAMAT): An open-label, randomised trial. *Lancet.* 2010;376(9753):1647–1657. https://doi.org/10.1016/S0140-6736(10)61924-1

27

BPaL, A New Oral Regimen for Drug-Resistant Tuberculosis

The Nix-TB Study

TUSHAR GARG

[Extensive drug resistant] tuberculosis and complicated [multidrug-resistant] tuberculosis can be treated with a regimen consisting of three oral agents for 26 weeks. Despite these forms of tuberculosis being historically hard-to-treat conditions, treatment success was 90%. . . .[1]

Research Question: What is the efficacy, safety, side-effect profile, and pharmacokinetics of the BPaL regimen (bedaquiline [B], pretomanid [Pa], and linezolid [L]) for the treatment of multidrug-resistant tuberculosis (MDR-TB) and extensive drug-resistant tuberculosis (XDR-TB)?

Funding: TB Alliance (Global Alliance for TB Drug Development); UK Department for International Development, UK Department of Health; Bill and Melinda Gates Foundation; U.S. Agency for International Development; Directorate General for International Cooperation of the Netherlands; Irish Aid; Australia Department of Foreign Affairs and Trade; Federal Ministry for Education and Research of Germany; Medical Research Council; National Research Foundation of South Africa.

Year Study Began: 2015

Year Study Published: 2020

Study Location: 3 sites in South Africa: Sizwe Tropical Disease Hospital, Johannesburg; Task Applied Science at Brooklyn Chest Hospital, Cape Town; King DiniZulu Hospital Complex, Durban

Who Was Studied: Patients with pulmonary TB who were 14 years or older weighing 35 kg or more with XDR-TB *or* MDR-TB not responsive to treatment *or* MDR-TB where second-line regimen was discontinued after side effects.

Who Was Excluded: Patients not expected to survive beyond 12 weeks; HIV-infected individuals with CD4+ count of 50 cells/μL or fewer; grade 3 or 4 peripheral neuropathy.

How Many Patients: 109 (XDR: 79, MDR: 38).

Study Overview: See Figure 27.1.

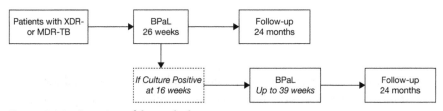

Figure 27.1. Overview of the study design.

Study Intervention: In this Phase 3, open-label study, patients with XDR-TB and complicated MDR-TB received BPaL regimen for 26 weeks. BPaL consisted of bedaquiline (400 mg once daily for 2 weeks, followed by 200 mg thrice per week), pretomanid (200 mg daily for 26 weeks), linezolid (1200 mg for up to 26 weeks, with dose adjustment permitted based on toxic adverse effects). Treatment could be extended to 39 weeks for patients with a positive culture at 16 weeks.

Follow-Up: 24 months

Endpoints:
  Primary endpoint: Incidence of an unfavorable outcome—clinical or bacteriological treatment failure *or* relapse—through follow-up until 6 months after the end of treatment.
  Secondary endpoint: Time to an unfavorable outcome, time to sputum culture conversion, all-cause mortality, incidence of adverse events that occurred or worsened during treatment.

RESULTS

- In intention-to-treat analysis, 11 (10%) of 109 enrolled patients had an unfavorable outcome at 6 months after treatment completion. Of the 11, 7 patients died, 1 withdrew consent, 2 relapsed, and 1 was lost to follow-up.
- Overall, 90% (95% CI 83–95, $n = 98$) of patients had a favorable outcome, defined as resolution of clinical disease, negative culture status, and not being classified as having had an unfavorable outcome (see Table 27.1).
- 17% of patients had a serious adverse event; 81% and 48% of patients developed peripheral neuropathy and myelosuppression, respectively.

Table 27.1 EFFICACY OF BPaL REGIMEN

Primary outcome	XDR ($n = 71$)	MDR ($n = 38$)	Overall ($n = 109$)
Proportion with favorable outcome (95% CI)	89% (79–95)	92% (79–98)	90% (83–95)

Criticisms and Limitations:

- This was a single group study instead of a randomized controlled trial. Efficacy estimates cannot be compared in the absence of a control arm. Nonetheless, results of this study are impreffive and significant given the prevailing high mortality and poor treatment outcomes in this form of TB.
- These results have limited generalizability because the study was conducted in a single country with a distinct TB and HIV epidemiology. Even though results are impressive, the stringent inclusion criteria mean that study patients may not be representative of the general population who could benefit from this regimen.[1,2]

Other Relevant Studies and Information:

- MDR-TB and XDR-TB treatment is a fast-developing field with several ongoing trials which will result in continual updates to the treatment guidelines and standards of care.

- Unpublished study completion results from the Nix-TB study report sustained favorable outcomes (88% in intention-to-treat analysis) with improvement in linezolid-induced peripheral neuropathy over 24 months post-treatment follow-up.[3]
- ZeNix trial, a follow-up to Nix-TB study, is underway to test alternative doses and durations of linezolid in the BPaL regimen for XDR-TB and complicated MDR-TB patients.[4] Early unpublished results report high treatment success rate with a lower dosage of linezolid and fewer adverse effects.[5]
- TB-PRACTECAL, a multi-country, Phase 2–3, randomized trial testing an all-oral regimen for MDR-TB patients ended its enrollment early in February 2021 based on the promising interim results.[6] Phase 3 was testing a 6-month regimen of BPaL + moxifloxacin versus country-specific standard of care, in which the former was superior to the control arm according to the unpublished results.[7]
- The World Health Organization (WHO) issued a rapid communication on the guidance to treat drug-resistant TB. The updates include a shorter regiment of 6 months of all-oral regimen of BPaL with or without moxifloxacin.[8]

Summary and Implications: The all-oral, 6-month BPaL regimen for patients with XDR-TB and complicated MDR-TB was highly effective in this single-group study. While the treatment regimen utilized in this study is easier and shorter compared to prior regimens, the incidence and severity of adverse effects caused by linezolid raise concerns about its broad applicability. Based on these results, the WHO has issued a rapid communication to use this regimen. The forthcoming results of ZeNix and TB-PRACTECAL trials will strengthen the evidence base and potentially offer solutions to the problem of high adverse events and side effects.

PROGRAMMATIC AND POLICY CASE: IMPLEMENTATION OF MDR AND XDR-TB TREATMENT PROGRAM

Case Overview

A low- and middle-income country with a high TB burden is worried about the increasing incidence of MDR-TB and XDR-TB. Several members raised this problem, along with that of poor treatment outcome and high mortality, in a parliamentary session, upon which the government instituted a high-level committee with diverse expertise to suggest a plan of action. A consultant excited by the recently published Nix-TB study brings forth the proposal to introduce BPaL into the national TB program to the committee. Looking for an immediate solution, the committee is inclined to make it one of the top priorities. As the resident public health expert on the committee, what do you advise the committee members?

Suggested Answer

The Nix-TB evidence is indeed impressive. However, the evidence should be evaluated carefully and contextualized before it is incorporated into TB programs. It was a single-group study without randomization or a control group. The aim was to evaluate the safety and efficacy of this novel regimen in XDR-TB and complicated MDR-TB patients. Robust evidence from randomized controlled trials (RCTs) is required before BPaL regimen can be included in treatment modalities.

While 90% of patients had a favorable outcome in Nix-TB, the high incidence and severity of adverse effects in the study cannot be sidelined. In a trial setting, careful measures are taken to record and manage adverse events and side effects. Further, it is distinct from a routine setting in terms of patient profile and diversity, and availability of resources and specialized personnel. Even if RCTs support the high efficacy, implementing the BPaL regimen will require implementation capacity assessment and provision of adverse events and side effects monitoring and management, both of which are sparse in a low-resource setting.

These limitations do not mean that the country should not prepare for newer regimens which have shown promise in the Nix-TB and other ongoing trials. Clinical and programmatic implementation will require context-specific evidence for introduction and scale-up of new treatment modalities for XDR-TB and MDR-TB. BPaL regimen can be introduced in an operational research setting—also recommended by the WHO—to supplement current evidence on efficacy and safety, and to build a localized understanding of implementation challenges and required resources.[8]

References

1. Conradie F, Diacon AH, Ngubane N, et al. Treatment of highly drug-resistant pulmonary tuberculosis. *N Engl J Med.* 2020;382(10):893–902. doi:10.1056/NEJMoa1901814

2. Global Alliance for TB Drug Development. *A Phase 3 Open-Label Trial Assessing the Safety and Efficacy of Bedaquiline Plus PA-824 Plus Linezolid in Subjects with Pulmonary Infection of Either Extensively Drug-Resistant Tuberculosis (XDR-TB) or Treatment*

Intolerant/Non-Responsive Multi-Drug Resistant Tuberculosis (MDR-TB). clinicaltrials. gov; 2020. Accessed September 30, 2021. https://clinicaltrials.gov/ct2/show/NCT0 2333799

3. Conradie F, Diacon A, Ngubane N, et al. Final results of the Nix-TB clinical study of BPaL regimen for highly resistant TB. In: *The Conference on Retroviruses and Opportunistic Infections (CROI)*; 2021. Abstract 562; Tuberculosis Prevention and Treatment; Accessed October 1, 2021. https://www.croiconference.org/abstract/ final-results-of-the-nix-tb-clinical-study-of-bpal-regimen-for-highly-resistant-tb/

4. Global Alliance for TB Drug Development. *A Phase 3 Partially-Blinded, Randomized Trial Assessing the Safety and Efficacy of Various Doses and Treatment Durations of Linezolid Plus Bedaquiline and Pretomanid in Participants with Pulmonary Infection of Either Extensively Drug-Resistant Tuberculosis (XDR-TB), Pre-XDR-TB or Treatment Intolerant or Non-Responsive Multi-Drug Resistant Tuberculosis (MDR-TB)*. clinicaltrials. gov; 2021. Accessed September 30, 2021. https://clinicaltrials.gov/ct2/show/NCT0 3086486

5. Conradie F, Everitt D, Olugbosi M, et al. High rate of successful outcomes treating highly resistant TB in the ZeNix study of pretomanid, bedaquiline and alternative doses and durations of linezolid. *J Int AIDS Soc.* 2021;24:70–71. Accessed October 1, 2021. https://go.gale.com/ps/i.do?p=HRCA&sw=w&issn=17582652&v=2.1&it= r&id=GALE%7CA672359471&sid=googleScholar&linkaccess=abs

6. Médecins Sans Frontières, Netherlands. *A Randomised, Controlled, Open-Label, Phase II–III Trial to Evaluate the Safety and Efficacy of Regimens Containing Bedaquiline and Pretomanid for the Treatment of Adult Patients with Pulmonary Multidrug Resistant Tuberculosis*. clinicaltrials.gov; 2021. Accessed September 30, 2021. https://clinicaltri als.gov/ct2/show/NCT02589782

7. Nyang'wa B-T, Motta I, Kazounis E, Berry C. Early termination of randomisation into TB-PRACTECAL, a novel six months all-oral regimen Drug Resistant TB study. *J Int AIDS Soc.* 2021;24:70–71. Accessed October 1, 2021. https://go.gale.com/ps/ i.do?p=AONE&sw=w&issn=17582652&v=2.1&it=r&id=GALE%7CA672359 470&sid=googleScholar&linkaccess=abs

8. Rapid communication: Key changes to the treatment of drug-resistant tuberculosis. World Health Organization. 2022. Accessed June 20, 2022. https://www.who.int/ publications/i/item/WHO-UCN-TB-2022-2.

9. World Health Organization. *WHO Operational Handbook on Tuberculosis: Module 4: Treatment: Drug-Resistant Tuberculosis Treatment*. World Health Organization; 2020. Accessed October 1, 2021. https://apps.who.int/iris/handle/10665/332398

28

Can Household Contact Investigation Reduce Tuberculosis?

BHAVNA SETH

> Household-contact investigation plus standard passive case finding was more effective than standard passive case finding alone for the detection of tuberculosis. . . .[1]

Research Question: Is tuberculosis (TB) household-contact investigation effective, compared with standard, passive measures, in Vietnam?

Funding: Australian National Health and Medical Research Council; ACT2 Australian New Zealand Clinical Trials Registry number, ACTRN12610000600044.

Study Began and Conducted: October 2010–June 2015

Study Published: January 2018

Study Location: 8 out of 64 provinces in Vietnam. The 8 provinces had 112 districts, out of which 70 districts were selected for the study. Each district has an average population of approximately 500 000 in urban areas and 100 000 in rural areas, including the two largest cities (Hanoi and Ho Chi Minh City).

Who Was Studied: Index patients with TB were 15 years of age or older, had smear-positive pulmonary TB, and had attended the TB clinic in the selected district.

Who Was Excluded: Patients with no contacts in their household

How Many Patients: 10 964 index patients and 25 707 contacts

Study Overview: See Figure 28.1.

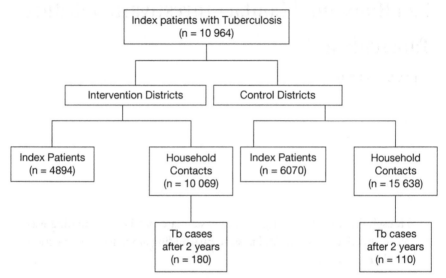

Figure 28.1. Overview of the study design.

Study Intervention: The 70 districts were the units of randomization in this cluster randomized controlled study. The combined population of the selected districts was 15 849 559 (18% of the Vietnamese population). Out of the 70 districts, 36 were intervention districts and 34 were control districts.

Contacts who were enrolled in intervention districts were given written information about TB and were invited to attend screening at the district clinic at enrollment and then at 6, 12, and 24 months. While contacts of control clinics were not screened, they completed a questionnaire and were asked to return after 24 months.

Follow-Up: 24 months

Endpoints:
   Primary study outcome: The proportion of contacts who were registered as having TB by the National Tuberculosis Program.
   Secondary outcomes: The number of persons in whom TB was confirmed on the basis of smear, culture, or polymerase-chain reaction assay, as well as all-cause mortality.

RESULTS

- From October 2010 through June 2013, 10 964 index patients and 25 707 contacts were enrolled.
- During the 2-year follow-up period, 180 contacts (1788 per 100 000 population) were registered as having TB in the intervention districts, as compared with 110 contacts (703 per 100 000 population) in the control districts.
- After adjustment for prior treatment, the relative risk of being listed in the TB registry was 2.6 (95% CI 2.0 to 3.3) in intervention districts, as compared with control districts.
- The number of persons who would need to be screened to gain one additional registered case of TB was 74.6 (95% CI, 64.2 to 89.2).
- Smear-positive TB was significantly more common among contacts in the intervention districts than in the control districts (relative risk, 6.4; 95% CI 4.5 to 9.0; p <0.001)
- In post hoc analyses, death from any cause was reported in 60 of 10 069 contacts (0.6%) in the intervention districts and in 265 of 15 638 contacts (1.7%) in the control districts (relative risk, 0.60; 95% CI 0.50 to 0.80; p <0.001)
- More than 95% of all household contacts of index cases in this study who received a diagnosis of incident TB were older than 15 years of age.

Table 28.1 SUMMARY OF KEY FINDINGS

Timing of diagnosis	Intervention Districts ($n = 10\ 069$)		Control Districts ($n = 15\ 638$)	
	Contacts with symptoms	Contacts with radiographic abnormalities	Contacts with registered case of TB	Contacts with registered case of TB
At any visit	1384/10 069 (13.7)	906/10 069 (9.0)	180/10 069 (1.8)	110/15 638 (0.7)
At baseline visit	667/10 069 (6.6)	344/10 069 (3.4)	48/10 069 (0.5)	NA
Between baseline and 6 months	69/10 069 (0.7)	47/10 069 (0.5)	21/10 069 (0.2)	44/15 638 (0.3)
At 6-month visit	221/6645 (2.2)	170/6645 (2.6)	34/6645 (0.5)	NA
Between 6 and 12 months	28/10 069 (0.3)	25/10 069 (0.2)	12/10 069 (0.1)	14/15 638 (0.1)
At 12 months	180/5644 (3.2)	142/5644 (2.5)	30/5644 (0.5)	NA
Between 12 and 24 months	57/10 069 (0.6)	47/10 069 (0.5)	14/10 069 (0.1)	52/15 638 (0.3)
At 24-month visit	162/7388 (2.2)	131/7388 (1.8)	21/7388 (0.3)	NA

Criticisms and Limitations: Average household size in the control districts was higher than intervention districts (3.9 persons vs. 3.3 persons), and a lower proportion of contacts in the control districts reported a prior history of TB (1.9% vs. 2.7%). These differences may have confounded the results.

Other Relevant Studies and Information:

- An economic evaluation of this trial was performed to understand the costs and cost effectiveness of active case finding. Healthcare costs were determined with a standardized national costing survey. The incremental cost effectiveness ratio per DALY averted was US$544. Active case finding was shown to be highly cost-effective in a setting with a high prevalence of TB.[2]
- In 2018, WHO made recommendation for TB preventive therapy for all household contacts exposed to a patient with TB even in high TB prevalence settings after ruling out active TB.[3]
- A study based on this recommendation by Paradkar et al. also suggests that TB preventive treatment should be offered to all household contacts of pulmonary TB patients residing in a high TB burden country such as India.[4]

Summary and Implications: This large, cluster-randomized, controlled pragmatic trial, conducted across 70 districts in Vietnam, demonstrated that household contact investigation plus passive case finding is more effective than passive case finding alone for managing TB in high-prevalence settings.

CLINICAL CASE: HOLISTIC MANAGEMENT OF TUBERCULOSIS

Case History
You are a community health worker, working in Rwanda. A 54-year-old farmer recently has been diagnosed with TB in your district health center. What should you counsel and arrange for him and for his family? What do the data suggest for treatment for his family? How long should you monitor his family?

Suggested Answer
At the outset, the family should be counseled about the infectiousness of TB, and its mechanisms of spread, and compounding factors—such as poor

nutrition and immunodeficiency diseases like diabetes mellitus and HIV. Similarly, household contacts with risk factors and children should be screened. Counseling should be done in a safe space with respect, with mitigation of concerns for stigma in the community. According to the local system, the patient should enroll, and follow up with TB treatment. The family members, or close contacts, should also have symptom screens at diagnosis, and should be counseled on further suggestive signs of TB to seek early care and treatment. Reassurance about treatment outcomes and setting expectations about what treatment entails should be provided. While Dr. Fox's trial suggests 2 years of follow-up, the extent of follow-up is to be determined, and may be longer. Further, the ability to test contacts for latent TB and to provide treatment is imperative per evolving evidence; however, implementation and uptake are per local guidelines, balanced by concerns for drug-resistant TB.

References

1. Fox GJ, Nhung NV, Sy DN, et al. Household-contact investigation for detection of tuberculosis in Vietnam. *N Engl J Med*. 2018 Jan 18;378(3):221–229. doi: 10.1056/NEJMoa1700209. PMID: 29342390.

2. Lung T, Marks GB, Nhung NV, et al. Household contact investigation for the detection of tuberculosis in Vietnam: economic evaluation of a cluster-randomised trial. *Lancet Glob Health*. 2019 Mar;7(3):e376–e384. doi: 10.1016/S2214-109X(18)30520-5. PMID: 30784638.

3. WHO. *Global Tuberculosis Report Geneva*. World Health Organization; 2018. https://apps.who.int/iris/bitstream/handle/10665/274453/9789241565646-eng.pdf?ua=1.

4. Paradkar M, Padmapriyadarsini C, Jain D, et al.; CTRIUMPH-RePORT India Study Team. Tuberculosis preventive treatment should be considered for all household contacts of pulmonary tuberculosis patients in India. *PLoS One*. 2020 Jul 29;15(7):e0236743. doi: 10.1371/journal.pone.0236743. PMID: 32726367; PMCID: PMC7390377

29

Solidarity Trial

The Dawn of a New Era

ANUP AGARWAL

> The main outcomes of mortality, initiation of ventilation, and hospitalization duration were not definitely reduced by any trial drug, either overall or in any particular subgroup.[1]

Research Question: Comparison of in-hospital mortality in patients with COVID-19 receiving local standard of care alone versus local standard plus either remdesivir or hydroxychloroquine (HCQ) or lopinavir/ritonavir or lopinavir/ritonavir with ionterferon.

Funding: The World Health Organization (WHO) was the global co-sponsor and national governments were national co-sponsors. Drugs were donated by pharmaceutical companies including Gilead Sciences, Mylan, AbbVie, Cipla, Merck, and Faron Pharmaceuticals.

Year Study Began: March 2020

Year Study Ended: October 2020

Study Location: 405 hospitals in 30 countries in all 6 WHO regions.

Who Was Studied: Patients above 18 years of age, hospitalized with a diagnosis of COVID-19, not known to have received any trial drug, not expected to be transferred elsewhere within 72 hours.

Who Was Excluded: Patients with contraindications to any of the available study drugs as per the randomizing clinicians.

How Many Patients Overall: 11 330 patients.

Study Overview: The Solidarity Trial was a large, international, adaptive, open-label, randomized controlled trial involving hospitalized participants to evaluate the effects of multiple repurposed drugs on mortality due to COVID-19 (see Figure 29.1).

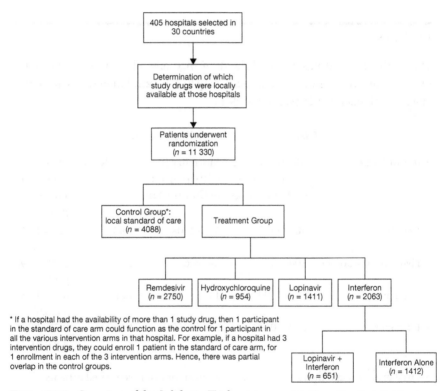

Figure 29.1. Overview of the Solidarity Trial.

Study Intervention: The regimen for remdesivir was 200 mg intravenous on day 0 and 100 mg once daily for 9 more days. The regimen for HCQ was 800 mg at hour 0, 800 mg at hour 6, and then starting at hour 12, 400 mg twice daily for 10 days. The regimen for lopinavir was 2 tablets twice daily for 14 days. The regimen for interferon was 44 micrograms on days 0, 3, and 6.

As Solidarity is an adaptive platform, currently, the 4 aforementioned drugs have been dropped as there was no benefit seen. In the same platform, now called

Solidarity Plus, 3 new additional drugs will be studied: artesunate, infliximab, and imatinib.

Follow-Up: Until discharge from hospital or death.

Endpoints:
The primary outcome was in-hospital mortality among all randomly assigned patients.
The secondary outcome was mechanical ventilation and time to discharge.

RESULTS

Out of the 4 trial drugs, none of the drugs had any effect on mortality, either overall or in any subgroup defined according to age, ventilation status at entry, or any other characteristics (see Table 29.1).

Table 29.1 SUMMARY OF KEY FINDINGS

Name of Drug	Mortality Rate of Participants on Study drugs	Mortality Rate of Participants in Control Arm	Rate Ratio	95% Confidence Interval; p Value
1. Remdesivir	301/2743	303/2708	0.95	0.81–1.11; $p = 0.50$
2. Hydroxychloroquine	104/947	84/906	1.19	0.89–1.59; $p = 0.23$
3. Lopinavir	148/1399	147/1372	1.00	0.79–1.25; $p = 0.97$
4. Interferon	243/2050	216/2050	1.16	0.96–1.39; $p = 0.11$

No trial drug reduced the initiation of ventilation among non-ventilated patients.

Criticisms and Limitations: The main criticism of an open label design is the risk of interviewer or physician bias, especially while evaluating subjective clinical improvement, the outcomes of which may be affected by the physician knowing the allocation of the patient.

Other Relevant Studies and Information:

- The Adaptive COVID-19 Trial was a double-blind, randomized, placebo-controlled trial that showed a shorter median time to discharge from randomization in patients receiving remdesivir (10 days with remdesivir versus 15 days with placebo).[2] However, the Solidarity Trial had a much larger sample size than the Adaptive COVID-19 Trial, and the latter study had a larger number of patients in the control arm requiring supplemental oxygen.
- The most important strength of the Solidarity Trial was its simplicity and the adaptive nature of the trial, allowing the simultaneous testing of 4 important therapeutic modalities. As such, this trial provided a swift answer during a global crisis. Similar simple, large-scale, adaptive studies were also done, such as the RECOVERY Trial[3] in the United Kingdom and DisCoVeRy Trial,[4] among many others. The RECOVERY trial provided important insights regarding the efficacy of steroids and tocilizumab in COVID-19, while the DisCoVeRy Trial showed there was no efficacy of remdesivir in patients hospitalized with COVID-19.

Summary and Implications: The Solidarity Trial was a simple, high-quality, global trial which swiftly provided insights on the efficacy of several drug treatments during the COVID-19 pandemic. The trial demonstrated that remdesivir, hydroxychloroquine (HCQ), lopinavir/ritonavir, and lopinavir/ritonavir with interferon were not efficacious in reducing mortality in patients hospitalized with COVID-19. These results were especially relevant for low- and middle-income countries for ensuring that scarce resources were not allocated to expensive, ineffective therapies.

POLICY CASE: IMPLEMENTATION OF AN ADAPTIVE TRIAL

Case Overview
You are the clinical trial expert on infectious diseases at the WHO Southeast Asia region. In the month of March, you convene over a meeting to discuss emerging therapeutics for dengue. In the meeting, based on consensus of experts, it is decided that there are 3 potential re-purposed therapies and one

new monoclonal antibody for dengue which are all deemed safe but efficacy has not been established.

As the clinical trial expert, how do you plan to approach this problem in the upcoming dengue season?

Suggested Answer

While there could be many ways to approach this complex problem, one solution based on the principles learned from the Solidarity Trial is as follows: dengue is a seasonal disease with wide geographical distribution across the Southeast Asia region. It is not possible to predict where dengue disease will cause higher case loads, as well as the severity of disease.

Based on this information, and the availability of 4 potential therapeutics, an adaptive randomized clinical trial of the 4 drugs across the Southeast Asia region, involving a large number of hospitals to ensure enrollment of a large number of participants, may be a sound approach, even if the disease spread is limited to certain geography. Such an approach may be helpful in assessing the efficacy of 4 potential therapeutic options.

Because the important outcome in an infectious disease like dengue is mortality, a simple trial looking at a specific outcome which can be conducted at a large scale will be of more value in comparison to a smaller trial assessing multiple outcomes and answering many questions.

References

1. WHO Solidarity Trial Consortium, Pan H, Peto R, Henao-Restrepo AM, et al. Repurposed antiviral drugs for COVID-19: Interim WHO Solidarity Trial Results. *N Engl J Med.* 2021 Feb 11;384(6):497–511. doi: 10.1056/NEJMoa2023184. PMID: 33264556; PMCID: PMC7727327.
2. Beigel JH, Tomashek KM, Dodd LE, et al.; ACTT-1 Study Group Members. Remdesivir for the treatment of COVID-19: Final report. *N Engl J Med.* 2020 Nov 5;383(19):1813–1826. doi: 10.1056/NEJMoa2007764. PMID: 32445440; PMCID: PMC7262788.
3. RECOVERY Collaborative Group, Horby P, Lim WS, Emberson JR, et al. Dexamethasone in hospitalized patients with COVID-19. *N Engl J Med.* 2021 Feb 25;384(8):693–704. doi: 10.1056/NEJMoa2021436. PMID: 32678530; PMCID: PMC7383595.
4. Ader F, Bouscambert-Duchamp M, Hites M, et al.; DisCoVeRy Study Group. Remdesivir plus standard of care versus standard of care alone for the treatment of patients admitted to hospital with COVID-19 (DisCoVeRy): A phase 3, randomised, controlled, open-label trial. *Lancet Infect Dis.* 2022 Feb;22(2):209–221. doi: 10.1016/S1473-3099(21)00485-0. PMID: 34534511; PMCID: PMC8439621.

30

Corticosteroids for Bacterial Meningitis in Adults in Sub-Saharan Africa

PRIYANK JAIN

Adjuvant therapy with dexamethasone for bacterial meningitis in adults from an area with a high prevalence of HIV did not reduce mortality or morbidity.[1]

Research Question: In patients hospitalized for suspected acute bacterial meningitis, does addition of systemic corticosteroids, along with systemic antibiotics, improve clinical outcomes?

Funding: Meningitis Research Foundation, UK, and pharmaceutical companies that manufacture ceftriaxone and dexamethasone used in the study.

Year Study Began: 2002–2005

Year Study Published: 2007

Study Location: A university teaching hospital in Malawi

Who Was Studied: Patients older than 16 years with clinical suspicion for bacterial meningitis and cerebrospinal fluid (CSF) findings consistent with bacterial meningitis. The findings could be grossly cloudy fluid, neutrophilic leukocytosis, or positive Gram's stain on microscopy.

Who Was Excluded: Patients who received corticosteroids for another reason, cryptococcus or tuberculosis detected on microscopy, or contraindications to the study drugs.

How Many Patients: 465 patients.

Study Overview: See Figure 30.1.

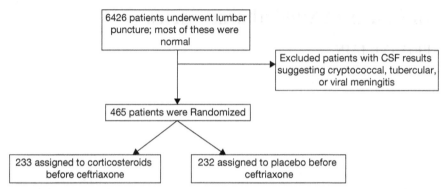

Figure 30.1. Overview of the study design.

Study Intervention: Dexamethasone 16 mg twice daily intravenously for 4 days, administered immediately before administration of ceftriaxone (2 g twice daily for 10 days).

Follow-Up: Treated in hospital for a minimum of 10 days and evaluated at 40 days and 6 months. Outcome at 40 days was available for 99% of patients.

Endpoints: Primary outcome was mortality at 40 days. Secondary outcomes included hearing impairment at day 40.

RESULTS

- Demographic info: Mean age 32 years, median time to presentation was 72 hours, and GCS was 10–11; 90% were HIV positive with a median CD4 count of 102; 70% had proven bacterial meningitis and 22% probable bacterial. *S pneumoniae* was isolated in 60% of all patients. Almost a third had received antibiotics before enrollment.
- See Table 30.1 for study results.

Table 30.1 SUMMARY OF KEY FINDINGS

	Corticosteroid Group	Placebo Group	Odds Ratio
Death, day 40	129/231 (56%)	120/228 (53%)	Not significant
Hearing loss, day 40	30/96 (31%)	36/99 (36%)	Not significant

Criticism and Limitations:

- Almost 40% of patients had received antibiotics before enrolling in the trial and getting corticosteroids. This can reduce the beneficial effect of steroids. However, when analysis was restricted to patients who did not receive antibiotics before enrollment, there was still no difference in outcomes.
- The study population has a high prevalence of HIV (90%) and these patients were not on antiretroviral treatment. This is quite different from other trials[2,3] where the HIV prevalence is low and there was benefit seen from the adjuvant corticosteroids. Hence, the negative results should not be generalized to other African countries or populations where the HIV prevalence is low or where patients are on antiretroviral therapy (ART).

Other Relevant Studies and Literature:

- The rationale for corticosteroids is derived from experimental animal models of infection, where it is demonstrated that subarachnoid space inflammatory response during bacterial meningitis is a major factor contributing to morbidity and mortality. Use of corticosteroids for bacterial meningitis in humans has been a controversial topic for decades without high-quality placebo-controlled trials.
- In 2002, *The New England Journal of Medicine*[2] published a trial with 301 European adults with bacterial meningitis which showed that fewer patients in the dexamethasone group died or were disabled as compared with the placebo group.
- That same year, 2002, *Lancet*[4] published a trial with 598 Malawian children in Queen Elizabeth Central Hospital, which showed that dexamethasone had no effect on the rates of death or neurologic sequelae.

- Infectious Diseases Society of America (IDSA) guidelines have not been updated since 2004[5] and predate this trial. European Society of Clinical Microbiology and Infectious Diseases (ESCMID) guidelines of 2016[6] did not include this trial's results. Both these guidelines recommend use of dexamethasone in adults with acute bacterial meningitis, although the European guideline restricts it to high-income countries. World Health Organization (WHO) guidelines (2015)[7] for managing meningitis epidemics in Africa do not recommend use of adjuvant steroids.

Summary and Implications: This trial found that adjuvant therapy with corticosteroids in adults with bacterial meningitis in an area with high prevalence of HIV did not reduce mortality or morbidity. The benefit of corticosteroids seen in studies from Europe and Vietnamese trials cannot be extrapolated to the settings with a high prevalence of HIV, such as sub-Saharan Africa.

CLINICAL CASE: MANAGEMENT OF MENINGITIS IN REGIONS WITH HIGH PREVALENCE OF HIV

Case History

You are working in a rural hospital in Malawi and are evaluating a 30-year-old previously healthy woman with 2 days of high fever, headache, seizure, and altered consciousness. You suspect meningitis, and lumbar puncture shows 500 WBC/ml with 90% neutrophils, and gram positive diplococci. Will you give adjuvant dexamethasone with antibiotics in this case?

Suggested Answer

This patient has features consistent with acute bacterial meningitis. She matches the study population where use of adjunctive steroids was not beneficial. However, unlike the study population where 90% of patients had untreated HIV, this is a previously healthy person. The current trial did not have sufficient power to detect a treatment effect on patients without HIV. As such, this patient may resemble more closely the study population of trials in Europe[2] and Vietnam,[3] where a mortality benefit was seen among patients with proven bacterial meningitis in a low HIV prevalence area. I would recommend giving this individual adjuvant corticosteroids based on careful application of the current evidence.

References

1. Scarborough M, Gordon SB, Whitty CJ, et al. Corticosteroids for bacterial meningitis in adults in sub-Saharan Africa. *N Engl J Med.* 2007;357(24):2441–2450. doi:10.1056/NEJMoa065711

2. de Gans J, van de Beek D; European Dexamethasone in Adulthood Bacterial Meningitis Study Investigators. Dexamethasone in adults with bacterial meningitis. *N Engl J Med.* 2002;347(20):1549–1556. doi:10.1056/NEJMoa021334

3. Nguyen TH, Tran TH, Thwaites G, et al. Dexamethasone in Vietnamese adolescents and adults with bacterial meningitis. *N Engl J Med.* 2007;357(24):2431–2440. doi:10.1056/NEJMoa070852

4. Molyneux EM, Walsh AL, Forsyth H, et al. Dexamethasone treatment in childhood bacterial meningitis in Malawi: a randomised controlled trial. *Lancet.* 2002;360(9328):211–218. doi:10.1016/s0140-6736(02)09458-8

5. van de Beek D, Cabellos C, Dzupova O, et al. ESCMID guideline: Diagnosis and treatment of acute bacterial meningitis. *Clin Microbiol Infect.* 2016;22 Suppl 3:S37–S62. doi:10.1016/j.cmi.2016.01.007

6. Tunkel AR, Hartman BJ, Kaplan SL, et al. Practice guidelines for the management of bacterial meningitis. *Clin Infect Dis.* 2004;39(9):1267–1284. doi:10.1086/425368

7. World Health Organization. Managing meningitis epidemics in Africa. WHO publication; 2015. WHO reference number: WHO/HSE/GAR/ERI/2010.4 Rev.1.

31

Oral Maintenance Therapy for Cholera in Adults

PRANAB CHATTERJEE

The drastic reduction in the need for intravenous fluids which results from the use of an oral therapeutic solution should make it possible for cholera-treatment centers with limited supplies of intravenous fluids to reduce the mortality from cholera to a level previously not possible in the absence of abundant intravenous fluids.[1]

Research Question: Can the use of an oral therapeutic solution reduce the intravenous (IV) fluid requirement for adult patients suffering from cholera?

Funding: National Institutes of Health, Bethesda, USA, and the Pakistan-SEATO (Southeast Asia Treaty Organization) Cholera Research Laboratory

Year Study Began: Not specified, most likely 1967–1968

Year Study Published: August 1968

Study Location: Dacca, in the erstwhile East Pakistan, which is currently Dhaka, Bangladesh

Who Was Studied: 29 individuals, admitted to the wards of the Pakistan-SEATO Cholera Research Laboratory for cholera; ages ranged from 11 to 60 years.

Who Was Excluded: No explicit exclusion criteria were applied.

How Many Patients: 29

Study Overview: See Figure 31.1.

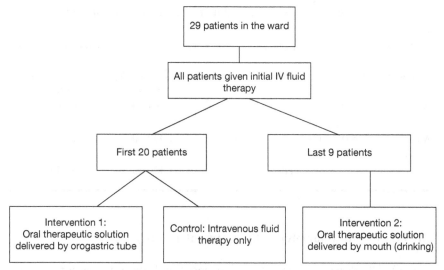

Figure 31.1. Overview of the study design.

Study Intervention: There were two intervention groups: the first group received oral therapeutic solution delivered by orogastric tube (the orogastric group), and the second group received the same solution per oral (by drinking). The control group received IV fluids.

In the orogastric fluid group, a solution containing electrolytes and glucose was delivered to the stomach via a thin orogastric tube. The control group received only IV fluids to compensate for stool losses. The second intervention group received the oral therapeutic solution delivered by mouth, that is, the patients drank the solution. Overall, there were 29 patients in the entire study.

All 29 patients received IV fluids initially, prior to being allocated to the three groups. All patients received 250 mg of tetracycline syrup once every 6 hours. All patients were prevented from taking anything else by mouth. Additional IV fluids were given to the oral fluid recipients to ensure that the specific gravity of their plasma did not exceed 1.030. Additional 25–50 ml of fluids were given by mouth to the recipients of the oral therapeutic solutions based on clinical judgment.

Follow-Up: Until diarrhea resolution

Endpoints: Amount of IV fluids needed by patients during the management of their cholera episode.

RESULTS

- There was a difference of nearly 15.5 L of total IV fluids needed between the oral therapy group and the IV fluid group, with the oral therapy group having a significantly smaller IV fluid requirement (see Table 31.1).

Table 31.1 ORAL VERSUS INTRA-VENOUS FLUID USE IN PATIENTS WITH CHOLERA

Characteristics	Oral Therapy Group	Intravenous Fluids Group
Mean volume of IV fluids given before allocation to oral or IV fluid groups	3494 ml	3400 ml
Mean volume of IV fluids given after allocation to oral or IV fluid groups	2000 ml	19 350 ml
Mean volume of IV fluids needed in total	4304 ml	19 800 ml

Adverse events associated with treatment groups:

- Oral fluids were remarkably well tolerated, and vomiting was not associated with receipt of oral fluids.
- The total volume of stool produced during the study period was significantly higher in the group receiving oral therapeutic fluids via orogastric tube, compared to the recipients of the IV therapy.
- Transient hypokalemia, associated with potassium losses in excessive diarrheal fluids, was observed in 5 of the 19 patients receiving oral fluids.
- Out of the 10 patients receiving fluids via the orogastric tube, 3 needed additional IV fluids; out of the 9 patients receiving fluids by mouth, 2 needed additional IV fluids.

Criticisms and Limitations:

- The study had a small sample size, which was not randomized to the 3 treatment groups. There were no mechanisms to ensure allocation concealment either. The sampling was purposive, and the study processes were also quite variable. This study was done before the current standards of quality expected from clinical trials became the norm.

Other Relevant Studies and Information:

- The major debate regarding oral rehydration solution (ORS) has been around using two different osmolarity solutions for cholera-associated diarrhea versus non-cholera-associated diarrhea. However, currently the World Health Organization (WHO) recommends a single osmolarity ORS for all causes of diarrhea. This ORS solution contains 75 meq of Na, 75 meq of glucose with total osmolarity of 245 mOsm/L. This reduced osmolarity ORS is as effective for cholera but is associated with higher risk of transient hyponatremia.

- This single osmolarity has been decided on the basis of the programmatic and logistical benefits of having a single ORS throughout the world and comparative efficacy of this solution for cholera-associated and non-cholera-associated diarrheal illness.[2]
- WHO recommends the use of IV fluids for the management of severe dehydration or shock in patients suffering from diarrhea.

Summary and Implications: Despite the significant methodological shortcomings, this study, conducted in the infancy of clinical trials, was instrumental in identifying the fact that if oral fluids were added to the management strategy for cholera, it would reduce the need for IV fluid support. This is especially significant because cholera is a bigger threat in resource-limited settings where oral fluids may be a more accessible treatment alternative.

CLINICAL CASE: ORT IN CHOLERA

Case History

A 26-year-old man is brought to the primary health center complaining of passing several episodes of watery stool. He does not report noticing any blood in the stool but does complain of colicky abdominal pain. He lives in a village which has recently reported several similar cases, which turned out to be cholera. Dark-field microscopy of the stool sample from this patient also shows *Vibrio* with darting motility, suggesting that he could be suffering from cholera. The patient is severely dehydrated and is slightly drowsy, but does mention that he feels very thirsty.

Based on the findings of this study, would you recommend adding oral therapeutic fluids after initial IV fluid resuscitation?

Suggested Answer

Given the initial finding of the patient being dehydrated, he needs IV fluids to replace the volume of fluids and electrolytes lost in the diarrheal fluids. Once the patient is resuscitated and is able to tolerate oral fluids, he can be shifted to receive oral fluids. Intravenous access should, however, be maintained if safe to do so, in case the patient needs additional IV fluids during the maintenance therapy period.

References

1. Nalin DR, Cash RA, Islam R, Molla M, Phillips RA. Oral maintenance therapy for cholera in adults. *Lancet*. 1968;2(7564):370–373. doi:10.1016/s0140-6736(68)90591-6
2. World Health Organization. Reduced osmolarity: Oral rehydration salts (ORS) formulation: A report from a meeting of experts jointly organised by UNICEF and WHO: UNICEF house, New York, USA, 18 July 2001. World Health Organization; 2002. Accessed October 25, 2021. https://apps.who.int/iris/handle/10665/67322.

SECTION 4

Child Health

Five studies were included in Section 4 on Child Health, though there is considerable overlap with other sections. As diarrheal illness is a major cause of morbidity and mortality in children worldwide, we included a study on zinc and diarrhea. Similarly, Helping Babies Breathe has been widely implemented at births. Bubble CPAP (continuous positive airway pressure) is one of the most common lifesaving strategies in pediatric intensive care units globally. We included the use of hydroxyurea in sickle cell disease because it is a life-altering intervention and highlights the population that suffers from this disease. The FEAST trial stresses, again, the fact that similar interventions may have varied outcomes depending on the clinical context.

Child Health

32

Efficacy of Zinc to Control Diarrhea in Developing Nations

COLLEEN KEOUGH

This study . . . documents the effectiveness of zinc supplementation as an adjunct to oral rehydration therapy and early continued feeding among preschool children with acute diarrhea.[1]

Research Question: What is the effect of zinc supplementation on the duration and severity of diarrhea?

Funding: Supported by the World Health Organization, Diarrheal Disease Control Program, the Thrasher Research Fund, and the Indian Council for Medical Research

Year Study Began: September 1992

Year Study Published: September 1995

Study Location: Kalkaji (neighborhood of New Delhi, India)

Who Was Studied: Patients of Kalkaji dispensary 6–35 months of age who were reported to have passed at least 4 unformed stools in the previous 24 hours and had diarrhea for less than 7 days. They were also required to be permanent residents of Kalkaji.

Who Was Excluded: Children who presented to the clinic a second time, were judged to have malnutrition requiring hospitalization, or whose parents did not consent.

How Many Patients: 947

Study Overview: See Figure 32.1.
- This was a double-blind randomized, controlled trial.
- A baseline assessment was performed by a research physician with measurements of height, length, and dehydration status and subsequently divided into smaller groups based on z-score (distance from the mean) and breastfeeding status. A venous blood sample was collected for estimation of zinc levels.
- Each participant was visited at home approximately every 5 days to collect data on stool output.

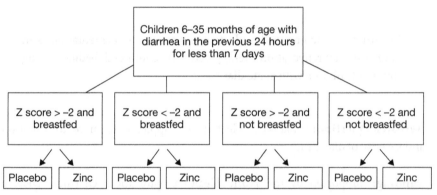

Figure 32.1. Summary of zinc supplementation in young children with acute diarrhea in India.

Study Intervention: Once randomized, each participant was given either a vitamin preparation with zinc gluconate (20 mg of elemental zinc) or a vitamin preparation with placebo.

Follow-Up: Every 5 days. After 10 days of diarrhea, children were given antibiotics.

Endpoints:
Primary outcome: Duration of diarrhea.
Secondary outcomes included diarrhea lasting more than 7 days from the start of treatment, mean number of watery stools per day, and visits to a physician.

RESULTS

- Supplementation with zinc was associated with a 23% reduction in risk of continued diarrhea.
- The relative risk of continued diarrhea in the zinc-supplementation group was 0.93 (95% CI 0.78–1.09) during days 1, 2, and 3, and 0.62 after day 3 (95% CI 0.52–0.73).
- The odds ratio for diarrhea lasting more than 7 days was 0.79 with zinc supplementation (95% CI 0.64–0.96).
- There was a 39% reduction in the mean number of watery stools per day and a 21% reduction in the number of days with watery stools.
- The mean number of watery stools per day was 3.1+/–9.9, as compared with 5.1+/–14.9 in the control group.
- Children with stunted growth had a greater reduction in watery stools 0.59 [95% CI 0.48–0.73] vs. 0.95 [95% CI 0.79–1.15]
- Among children with wasting (z-score weight for length < –2), the risk reduction was more significant (0.48; 95% CI 0.39–0.68).
- There were no significant differences related to plasma zinc levels or physician visits.
- Emesis occurred in an equal amount in both groups after consuming supplement (2 in each group).

Criticisms and Limitations: This study was done in a specific setting and may not be generalizable to all countries, all socioeconomic statuses of patients, and all pediatric hospitals. Zinc is likely more effective in children with stunted growth. This study did not show effectiveness in children with normal growth in subgroup analysis.

Other Relevant Studies and Information: Acute diarrhea remains a leading cause of childhood deaths, with up to 2.5 million deaths estimated annually among children below 5 years of age.[2] Zinc likely plays an important role in modulating the host resistance to infectious agents by improving the absorption of water and electrolytes, improves regeneration of the intestinal epithelium, increases the levels of brush border enzymes, and enhances the immune response, allowing for better clearance of the pathogens.[3] Multiple studies have shown that zinc supplementation decreases the duration of acute diarrhea by 11.5 hours and can prevent diarrhea.[4,5,6,7] This is especially true in children who are malnourished, where zinc supplementation may decrease diarrhea by 26 hours.[4]

As a result of these studies, the World Health Organization (WHO), UNICEF, and USAID recommend zinc salt along with low osmolarity oral rehydration solution (ORS), with reduced levels of glucose and salt during episodes of acute diarrhea to reduce the duration and severity of the episode.[8] In addition, they recommend continued zinc supplementation for 10–14 days to decrease the incidence of subsequent episodes of diarrhea in the following 2–3 months.

Summary and Implications: This study demonstrates that in pediatric populations likely to have a high prevalence of zinc deficiency and malnutrition, zinc supplementation during episodes of diarrhea may decrease the frequency and duration of diarrhea. For children with normal growth and nutrition, supplementation is still of unclear benefit.

CLINICAL CASE: DIARRHEA IN AN 18-MONTH-OLD WITH STUNTED GROWTH

Case History

An 18-month-old female presents with watery diarrhea for 3 days. She has been having 6 or more stools per day. Her mother has been breastfeeding her, but she has not been improving. Her weight for length z-score is –2. Her exam is notable for generalized malaise, sunken eyes, and sinus tachycardia. She is breathing comfortably and abdomen is soft, nondistended. She is appropriately responsive on neurologic examination. What therapies discussed in this chapter may be appropriate for this patient?

Suggested Answer

Given her malnourishment and acute diarrhea, 20 mg zinc supplementation daily for 10–14 days would be appropriate therapy for her, especially since the child is only in her first 3 days of illness. It is likely this will shorten this episode of diarrhea. Additionally, she would benefit from syringe feeding low osmolarity oral rehydration salts (for more information on ORS, see: https://rehydrate.org/ors/low-osmolarity-ors.htm).

References

1. Sazawal S, Black RE, Bhan MK, Bhandari N, Sinha A, Jalla S. Zinc supplementation in young children with acute diarrhea in India. *N Engl J Med*. 1995 Sep 28;333(13):839–844. doi: 10.1056/NEJM199509283331304. PMID: 7651474.

2. Kosek M, Bern C, Guerrant RL. The global burden of diarrhoeal disease, as estimated from studies published between 1992 and 2000. *Bull World Health Organ.* 2003;81(3):197–204.

3. Bajait C, Thawani V. Role of zinc in pediatric diarrhea. *Indian J Pharmacol.* 2011;43(3):232–235. doi: 10.4103/0253-7613.81495

4. Lazzerini M, Ronfani L. Oral zinc for treating diarrhoea in children. *Cochrane Database Syst Rev.* 2008 Jul 16;(3):CD005436. doi: 10.1002/14651858.CD005436.pub2. Update in: *Cochrane Database Syst Rev.* 2012;(6):CD005436. PMID: 18646129.

5. Patel A, Mamtani M, Dibley MJ, Badhoniya N, Kulkarni H. Therapeutic value of zinc supplementation in acute and persistent diarrhea: A systematic review. *PLoS One.* 2010 Apr 28;5(4):e10386. doi: 10.1371/journal.pone.0010386. PMID: 20442848; PMCID: PMC2860998.

6. Scrimgeour AG, Lukaski HC. Zinc and diarrheal disease: Current status and future perspectives. *Curr Opin Clin Nutr Metab Care.* 2008 Nov;11(6):711–717. doi: 10.1097/MCO.0b013e3283109092. PMID: 18827574.

7. Trivedi SS, Chudasama RK, Patel N. Effect of zinc supplementation in children with acute diarrhea: Randomized double blind controlled trial. *Gastroenterology Res.* 2009 Jun;2(3):168–174. doi: 10.4021/gr2009.06.1298. PMID: 27933128; PMCID: PMC5139709.

8. *WHO/UNICEF Joint Statement: Clinical Management of Acute Diarrhea. WHO/FCH/CAH/04.7.* World Health Organization; 2004 May.

33

Fluids in Pediatric Sepsis

Are the Recommendations in the Global North and Global South the Same? The FEAST Trial

JESSICA TOP

> The results do not support the routine use of bolus resuscitation in severely ill febrile children with impaired perfusion in African hospitals and also raise questions about its use in other settings.[1]

Research Question: What are the effects of resuscitation with bolus fluids in children with severe febrile illness and impaired perfusion in a resource-poor, malaria-endemic setting?

Funding: Medical Research Council, UK; Baxter Healthcare donated solutions.

Year Study Began: 2009

Year Study Ended: 2011

Study Location: Uganda, Kenya, Tanzania

Who Was Studied: Children 60 days–12 years old presenting with severe febrile illness with impaired consciousness, respiratory distress, or both, along with impaired perfusion, defined as a capillary refill time of 3 or more seconds, lower-limb temperature gradient, weak radial-pulse volume, or severe tachycardia (>180 beats per minute in children younger than 12 months of age, >160 beats per minute in children 1–5 years of age, or >140 beats per minute in children older than 5 years of age). Severe febrile illness included: severe malaria, sepsis, pneumonia, meningitis.

Who Was Excluded: Severe malnutrition, gastroenteritis, non-infectious causes of shock,

How Many Patients: 3170 enrolled: 29 with severe hypotension, 3141 without severe hypotension

Study Overview: See Figure 33.1.

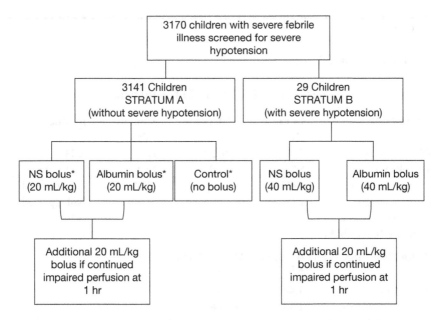

*If severe hypotension developed, the child was treated with 40 mL/kg boluses of study fluid (saline in the case of the control group)
Note: a protocol amendment increased initial boluses from 20 mL/kg in stratum A to 40 mL/kg, and from 40 mL/kg in stratum B to 60 mL/kg during the study

Figure 33.1. Overview of the study design.

Study Intervention: Patients were screened for hypotension. If normotensive, the patient was placed in Stratum A. If hypotensive, the patient was placed in Stratum B. In Stratum A, patients were randomized to receive a 20 mL/kg normal saline (NS) bolus, 20 mL/kg albumin bolus, or no bolus in the control group. Stratum B was randomized to receive a 40 mL/kg NS bolus or 40 mL/kg albumin bolus. Both groups received an additional 20 mL/kg at 1 hour if there was impaired perfusion. If a patient became hypotensive, 40 mL/kg of the groups' specified fluid was given, or 40 mL/kg normal saline in the control group.

Patients were given antimalarials, antibiotics, hypoglycemia treatment, anticonvulsants, as clinically appropriate. Blood transfusion was given if Hgb was <5 g/dL according to national guidelines. Authors state the timing of receipt of blood, quinine, and antibiotics were similar across all groups.

Follow-Up: 4 weeks

Endpoints: Death, pulmonary edema, increased Intracranial Pressure, severe hypotension, allergic reaction, pulmonary edema

RESULTS

See Tables 33.1 and 33.2.

Table 33.1 STRATUM A: 3141 CHILDREN

OUTCOME	Control (No bolus)	NS bolus	Albumin bolus	*p*-value
48-hour mortality	7.3%	10.5%	10.6%	.003
4-week mortality	8.7	12.0	12.2	.004
Pulmonary edema	0.6%	0.6%	1.3%	Not reported
Increased ICP	1.1%	1.7%	1.5%	Not reported
Pulmonary edema, increased ICP, or both	1.6%	2.2%	2.6%	.17

RELATIVE RISK (RR) OF DEATH AT 48 HOURS

Group	RR	*p*-value
NS vs. Control	1.44	.01
Albumin vs. Control	1.45	.008
Albumin vs. NS bolus	1.00	.96
Bolus vs. Control	1.45	.003

Table 33.2 STRATUM B: 29 CHILDREN

OUTCOME	NS bolus	Albumin bolus	*p*-value
Mortality	56%	69%	0.45

RELATIVE RISK OF DEATH AT 48 HOURS

Group	RR	*p*-value
Albumin vs NS	1.23	p = 0.45

- In Stratum A, both types of boluses significantly increased mortality at 48 hours and at 4 weeks.
  - Bolus resuscitation increased absolute risk of death at 48 hours by 3.3%.

- Risk of death was the same for all at 1 hour, then increased in the bolus groups.
- There was no significant increase of ICP or pulmonary edema in the bolus groups.
- At 48 hours in Stratum B, 56% of patients died in the NS group vs. 69% of patients in the albumin bolus group ($p = 0.45$).

Criticisms/Limitations:

- There is concern regarding the discrepancy in the inclusion criteria in the study protocol and the published paper. The original study protocol does not mention severe febrile illness as an inclusion criterion, but the amended protocol (June 2011) mentions severe febrile illnesses as an inclusion criterion.
- The parameters utilized to define hypovolemic shock in this study are not very specific.[2,3]
- It is possible that some children in the study had illnesses such as malaria that predispose to fluid overload and may be exacerbated by fluid boluses.[2,4]
- The FEAST findings may not be generalizable to contexts with different causes of shock and in centers with invasive monitoring, mechanical ventilation, and vasoactive drug infusions.

Other Relevant Studies and Information: The current standard of care for treating hypovolemic shock and impaired circulation are fluid boluses. Studies conducted in the Global North and well-resourced areas have shown that fluid resuscitation within the first hour improves survival rates,[5–7] and this was extrapolated to pediatric patients in a study of goal-directed therapy showing improved mortality and morbidity among children.[8]

However, as a result of the FEAST trial, the WHO suggests cautious fluid administration in children with malnourishment, anemia, or malaria, and the 2012 Surviving Sepsis campaign and American Heart Association recommend cautious fluid administration in children if there is limited access to critical care.[9,10]

Summary and Implications: The results of the FEAST trial suggest that fluids should be given cautiously in children 60 days–12 years old presenting with early signs of sepsis, particularly in resource-limited settings where access to critical care services is limited. This study suffers from methodological limitations, however, and more research is needed to better define the settings in which these findings apply.

CLINICAL CASE: DEHYDRATED 2-YEAR-OLD WITH FEVER

Case History

A 2-year-old girl presents to the emergency room in rural Liberia with a fever and decreased fluid intake over the past 2 days. She has had fever without cough, difficulty breathing, vomiting, or diarrhea. On exam she is listless in her father's arms. Her respiratory rate is 36/min, heart rate 166/min, blood pressure 86/60 mmHg, temperature 102.2°F, and oxygen saturation is 98% on room air. She has mucosal pallor noted on her tongue and conjunctiva. Mucosa is also dry. No respiratory distress, her lungs are clear. Her heart has a regular rate and rhythm, no murmurs. Abdomen soft, no hepatomegaly. No rash. Capillary refill is 4 sec. How should she be treated?

Suggested Answer

According to the results of the FEAST trial, this patient should not receive fluid resuscitation given the increase in mortality noted. However, given that she is tachypneic, tachycardic, hypotensive, and has delayed capillary refill in addition to mucosal pallor and dryness, there is evidence of septic shock. It stands to reason that given the significant limitations of this trial and poor inclusion criteria, she should still be treated with fluid resuscitation. Subsequently, laboratory tests to pursue a definitive diagnosis based on the major local epidemiological causes of febrile illness in this age group should be performed. In Liberia, one should consider malaria. However, treatment should also include empiric antibiotics based on local antibiotic practices, antipyretics, and supportive care.

References

1. Maitland K, Kiguli S, Opoka RO, et al.; FEAST Trial Group. Mortality after fluid bolus in African children with severe infection. *N Engl J Med*. 2011 Jun 30;364(26):2483–2495. doi: 10.1056/NEJMoa1101549. PMID: 21615299.
2. Southall D, Samuels M. Archives of disease in childhood. *BMJ*. 2011;96(10):905–906.
3. Tripathi A, Kabra SK, Sachdev HP, Lodha R. Mortality and other outcomes in relation to first hour fluid resuscitation rate: A systematic review. *Indian Pediatr*. 2015 Nov;52(11):965–972. doi: 10.1007/s13312-015-0754-3. PMID: 26615345.

4. Planche T, Onanga M, Schwenk A, et al. Assessment of volume depletion in children with malaria. *PLoS Med.* 2004;1(1):e18. doi:10.1371/journal.pmed.0010018

5. Carcillo JA, Davis AL, Zaritsky A. Role of early fluid resuscitation in pediatric septic shock. *JAMA.* 1991;266(9):1242–1245.

6. Han YY, Carcillo JA, Dragotta MA, et al. Early reversal of pediatric-neonatal septic shock by community physicians is associated with improved outcome. *Pediatrics.* 2003;112(4):793–799. doi:10.1542/peds.112.4.793

7. Rivers E, Nguyen B, Havstad S, et al. Early goal-directed therapy in the treatment of severe sepsis and septic shock. *N Engl J Med.* 2001;345(19):1368–1377. doi:10.1056/NEJMoa010307

8. de Oliveira CF, de Oliveira DS, Gottschald AF. ACCM/ PALS haemodynamic support guidelines for paediatric septic shock: An outcomes comparison with and without monitoring central venous oxygen saturation. *Intensive Care Med.* 2008;34:1065–1075.

9. Dellinger RP, Levy MM, Rhodes A, et al.; Surviving Sepsis Campaign Guidelines Committee including the Pediatric Subgroup. Surviving sepsis campaign: International guidelines for management of severe sepsis and septic shock: 2012. *Crit Care Med.* 2013;41:580–637.

10. Dewez JE, Nijman RG, Yeung S. Fluids in the management of sepsis in children: A review of guidelines in the aftermath of the FEAST trial. *Arch Dis Childhood.* 2019;104(12):1236. doi: http://dx.doi.org.liverpool.idm.oclc.org/10.1136/archdischild-2019-317595.

34

Does Helping Babies Breathe Training Help Reduce Neonatal Mortality?

SHEGUFTA SHEFA SIKDER

The [Helping Babies Breathe] approach is simple, emphasizing immediate drying and stimulation, an intervention that can be readily implemented at any delivery . . . to reduce early neonatal mortality.

—Neonatal mortality and fresh stillbirth rates in Tanzania after Helping Babies Breathe (HBB) training[1]

Research Question: Does implementation of the Helping Babies Breathe (HBB) program enhance the basic skills of birth attendants and reduce early neonatal mortality and rates of fresh stillbirth?

Funding: American Academy of Pediatrics & Laerdal Foundation for Acute Medicine

Year Study Began: September 2009–March 2012

Year Study Published: 2013

Study Location: 8 hospitals in Tanzania

Who Was Studied: All births for 2 months before and 2.5 years after implementation of the Helping Babies Breathe (HBB) program

Who Was Excluded: not applicable

How Many Patients: 86 624 (8124 births before implementation and 78 500 births after implementation)

Study Overview: See Figure 34.1.

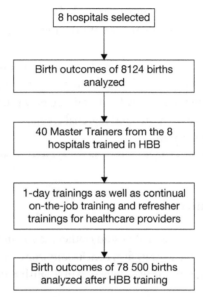

Figure 34.1. Overview of the study design.

Study Intervention: The HBB program emphasizes utilizing basic neonatal resuscitative steps, including drying, stimulating, and suctioning (if needed) to restore spontaneous respirations. First, there was a 2-day training of "master trainers" from the 8 hospitals included in the study. The research team and master trainers then conducted a 1-day training of healthcare providers at the sites, in addition to continual "on-the job" training and refresher trainings.

Follow-Up: Birth outcomes were recorded 2.5 years after implementation.

Endpoints: Reduction in early neonatal mortality (ENM) within 24 hours, rates of fresh stillbirths (FSB), and early perinatal mortality.

RESULTS

- HBB was associated with a 47% reduction in early neonatal mortality (ENM) within 24 hours (relative risk [RR] with training 0.53; 95% CI 0.43–0.65) and a 24% reduction in fresh stillbirths after 2 years (RR with training 0.76; 95% CI 0.64–0.90).

• The use of stimulation increased from 47% to 88% (RR 1.87; 95% CI 1.82–1.90) and suctioning increased from 15% to 22% (RR 1.40; 95% CI 1.33–1.46), whereas face mask ventilation decreased from 8.2% to 5.2% (RR 0.65; 95% CI 0.60–0.72).
• The significant reduction in ENM was observed in both term and preterm infants, and the positive impact extended to include those of lesser birth weight and gestational age with the highest inherent burden of death.
• This positive effect was achieved without supplemental oxygen in most cases, as well as endotracheal intubation or chest compressions.
• This study resulted in a "cascade" of training new trainers, and there is now a large core of master and regional trainers who have begun to disseminate the program.

Criticisms and Limitations:

• Since this was a before-and-after study rather than a randomized controlled trial, it is not possible to draw firm conclusions from this analysis.
• The intervention training was delivered in English rather than in the local language.

Other Relevant Studies and Information:

• While Helping Babies Breathe is an important intervention specific to neonatal mortality, the ability of the health facility to deliver these interventions depends on the strength of the wider health system to support training personnel initially and continually.[2,3] Other barriers to implementation include staff turnover and limited time or focus on training and practice. Post-training decline in knowledge and skills can be prevented with low-dose high-frequency refresher training, on-the-job practice, or similar interventions.[4]
• Researchers of several studies found HBB to be cost-effective.[5]
• A recent metanalysis[6] of 7 studies looking at the effect of HBB on neonatal outcomes showed moderate evidence for a decrease in intrapartum-related stillbirth and 1-day neonatal mortality rate after implementing the HBB training. However, to achieve an even greater effect, additional strategies (e.g., targeting temperature regulation) will likely be necessary to avoid later deaths. While this training package is a promising intervention specific to neonatal mortality, it is not

a catch-all intervention, as there are other major causes of neonatal mortality and threats to ill health among newborns and children which require wider systemic approaches.

Summary and Implications: The first day and especially the first hour is critical to newborn survival, with 60%–70% of neonatal deaths occurring in the first 24 hours. This study highlights the effectiveness of the HBB training and education curricula on neonatal mortality in under-resourced settings. The HBB approach is simple and can be implemented readily. A randomized trial would be required to confirm these encouraging results.

CLINICAL CASE: NEONATAL RESUSCITATION AT BIRTH

Case History
You are asked to help reduce early neonatal mortality in a rural district that consists of multiple health centers that have limited supplies, including no oxygen, and no electronic warmers. Based on this study, what interventions could you suggest to improve early neonatal mortality and fresh stillbirth?

Suggested Answer
As in this study, you could work with individuals from each health center to train them in the HBB curricula, focusing on stimulation, drying, and suctioning of babies to improve spontaneous respiration. You could encourage those trainers to train others at their healthcare facilities to induce this "cascading effect" of trainers and develop a cohort of well-trained individuals in basic neonatal resuscitation. Additionally, you should anticipate some of the barriers to implementation, including staff turnover and skill decline. With this in mind, determine ways to ensure that new staff arriving at health centers are trained in HBB, and ways to provide ongoing skills refreshers for current staff. Although HBB requires minimal resources, in order to properly perform HBB, you should make sure health centers have access to dry linens and suction bulbs.

References

1. Msemo G, Massawe A, Mmbando D, et al. Newborn mortality and fresh stillbirth rates in Tanzania after Helping Babies Breathe training. Pediatrics. 2013;131(2):e353–e360. doi: 10.1542/peds.2012-1795d

2. Senkubuge F, Modisenyane M, Bishaw T. Strengthening health systems by health sector reforms. *Glob Health Action.* 2014;7:23568. Published 2014 Feb 13. doi:10.3402/gha.v7.23568.
3. Swanson RC, Bongiovanni A, Bradley E, et al. Toward a consensus on guiding principles for health systems strengthening. *PLoS Med.* 2010 Dec;7(12):e1000385. doi: 10.1371/journal.pmed.1000385.
4. Morris S, Fratt E, Rodriguez J, Ruman A, Wibecan L, Nelson B. Implementation of the helping babies breathe training program: a systematic review. *Pediatrics.* 2020 Sep;146(3):e20193938.
5. Vossius C, Lotto E, Lyanga S, et al. Cost-effectiveness of the "Helping Babies Breathe" program in a missionary hospital in rural Tanzania. *PLoS One.* 2014;9(7):e102080.
6. Versantvoort JMD, Kleinhout MY, Ockhuijsen HDL, et al. Helping Babies Breathe and its effects on intrapartum-related stillbirths and neonatal mortality in low-resource settings: A systematic review. *Arch Dis Child.* 2020;105:127–133.

35

Bubble CPAP as a Cost-Effective Technology to Reduce Need for Mechanical Ventilation in Neonates

ANDREA WALKER

Safe mechanical ventilation requires a high level of expertise, and the constant availability of trained medical staff . . . it is highly advantageous if a simpler and cheaper intervention (bubble CPAP) can significantly reduce the need for mechanical ventilation with at least the same survival rate."

—KOYAMAIBOLE ET AL. 2005[1]

Research Question: Will the introduction of bubble continuous positive airway pressure (CPAP) affect neonatal case fatality rates in low-resource settings?

Funding: The Japanese Government Aid Organization

Year Study Began: 2001

Year Study Published: 2005

Study Location: Fiji

Who Was Studied: All neonates admitted to the NICU 18 months before and 18 months after the introduction of bubble CPAP in May 2003.

Who Was Excluded: None noted.

How Many Patients: 2488

Study Overview: See Figure 35.1.

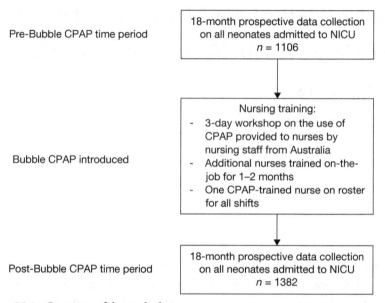

Figure 35.1. Overview of the study design.

Study Intervention: Before the intervention, nurses were limited to supplemental oxygen as their only treatment for neonates with respiratory distress. Mechanical ventilation was available, but could only be performed by a trained medical officer. Equipment was purchased to provide bubble CPAP to two neonates at any one time. Three senior nurses/midwives were trained to recognize babies in respiratory distress and to administer CPAP. A 3-day workshop on the use of CPAP was provided, and training of additional nurses was undertaken on the job for 1–2 months before a nurse was able to autonomously administer bubble CPAP. Each shift was staffed with a nurse trained in CPAP.

Follow-Up: 18 months

Endpoints: Neonatal mortality, need for any form of respiratory support, requirement for mechanical ventilation, requirement for bubble CPAP, requirement for mechanical ventilation after failing bubble CPAP.

RESULTS

- The baseline characteristics of the neonates requiring ventilatory support did not differ by mean weight or gestational age, but there were significantly more neonates weighing between 1000–1500g in the pre-bubble CPAP time period than the post-bubble CPAP time period (18.1% vs. 12.6%, respectively, $p = 0.008$).
- In the pre-bubble CPAP period, some form of respiratory support was required by 53.8% of neonates. In the post-bubble CPAP period, 40.2% of neonates required some form of respiratory support.
  - Mechanical ventilation requirements decreased by 50% once bubble CPAP was initiated, with 10.2% of neonates prior to bubble CPAP compared with 5.1% after bubble CPAP initiation ($p < 0.001$).
- There was no difference in mortality between the time periods when neonates requiring respiratory support were predominantly managed with mechanical ventilation (pre-bubble CPAP) and when they were predominantly managed with bubble CPAP (7.1% and 5.4% case fatality, respectively, $p = 0.065$) (see Table 35.1).

Table 35.1 Summary of the Study's Key Findings

Outcome	Pre-Bubble CPAP	Post-Bubble CPAP	p Value
Admitted to NICU	1106	1382	—
Some form of respiratory support needed	596 (53.8%)	556 (40.2%)	Not given
Need for mechanical ventilation	113 (10.2%)	70 (5.1%)	<0.001
Failed bubble CPAP and started mechanical ventilation	—	24	—
Neonatal death	79 (7.1%)	74 (5.4%)	0.065

Criticisms and Limitations:

- This was not a randomized trial, and as noted above, the weights of neonates born during the 2 time periods differed significantly for very low birth weight infants (1000–1500g) between the two analysis periods; this and other factors may have potentially confounded the results.

Other Relevant Studies and Information:

- CPAP is a non-invasive alternative form of respiratory support that is usually applied through a mechanical ventilator (ventilator-derived CPAP). Bubble CPAP is a cheaper and simpler way to administer CPAP without the use of mechanical ventilators. Additionally, bubble CPAP has several potential advantages over mechanical ventilation, including: lower cost, application by nursing staff, and lower risk of complications. As such, it has been proposed as an inexpensive method of delivering CPAP in developing countries.[2] It has been found to be fairly comparable to other forms of CPAP, and may actually lead to lower incidence of CPAP failure.[1,3,4]
- A systematic review of available literature similarly demonstrated that bubble CPAP can reduce the need for mechanical ventilation by 30%– 50% with no increase in mortality, echoing results shown in this study.[4]
- CPAP is strongly recommended by the World Health Organization (WHO) for the treatment of preterm newborns with respiratory distress syndrome, though this is contingent upon proper training and ability to monitor appropriately.[5]

Summary and Implications: In developing countries, bubble CPAP is safe and reduces the need for mechanical ventilation. Additionally, it is more affordable, less invasive, and can be applied and monitored by nursing staff after short training periods. As such, it is an excellent option for increasing available neonatal treatments for respiratory distress in low-resource settings.

CLINICAL CASE: STARTING AN NICU IN A LOW-RESOURCE SETTING

Case History

As part of the Ministry of Health in a rural district in a developing nation, you are asked for a plan to reduce neonatal mortality and are given a modest budget to start an NICU at the single district hospital, which has minimal physician staffing. The Ministry has already rolled out programs teaching basic neonatal resuscitation and has instituted the WHO Safe Childbirth Checklist at all health centers in the district, and at the district hospital. Using the information in this study and principles learned from other chapters, how might you consider approaching this problem?

Suggested Answer

Due to the cost and personnel constraints, an initial step in development of neonatal referral services could be the provision of bubble CPAP at the district hospital, rather than the use of mechanical ventilators. However, it is important to note that medical equipment alone does not constitute an NICU. Prior to undertaking this project, adequate initial neonatal care and initial referral-level care must be available, and effective transportation and communication systems must be in place. Programs to improve the general quality of neonatal care, monitoring, standardization of drug therapies, prevention of hypoglycemia and hypothermia, and peer review of outcomes are also essential components of referral-level neonatal care. Thought must be given to the required human and monetary resources for equipment upkeep and replacement parts. The study authors acknowledge that without addressing these issues "the impact of any form of respiratory support will be less than optimal."[3][1]

References

1. Koyamaibole L, Kado J, Qovu JD, Colquhoun S, Duke T. An evaluation of bubble-CPAP in a neonatal unit in a developing country: Effective respiratory support that can be applied by nurses. *J Trop Pediatr.* 2006 Aug;52(4):249–253. doi: 10.1093/tropej/fmi109. PMID: 16326752.
2. Upadhyay A, Deorari AK. Continuous positive airway pressure: A gentler approach to ventilation. *Indian Pediatr.* 2004;41:459–469.
3. Bharadwaj SK, Alonazi A, Banfield L, Dutta S, Mukerji A. Bubble versus other continuous positive airway pressure forms: a systematic review and meta-analysis. *Arch Dis Child Fetal Neonatal Ed.* 2020 Sep;105(5):526-531. doi: 10.1136/archdischild-2019-318165. PMID: 31969457.
4. Martin S, Duke T, Davis P. Efficacy and safety of bubble CPAP in neonatal care in low and middle income countries: A systematic review. *Arch Dis Child Fetal Neonatal Ed.* 2014 Nov 1;99(6):F495–F504.
5. WHO recommendations on interventions to improve preterm birth outcomes. WHO [Internet]. 2016 [cited 2023 Mar 14]. https://apps.who.int/iris/bitstream/handle/10665/183037/9789241508988_eng.pdf?sequence=1

36

Sickle Cell Anemia in Children in Sub-Saharan Africa—What Is the Best Medicine?

The REACH Trial

TIMOTHY S. LAUX

Hydroxyurea treatment was feasible and safe in children with sickle cell anemia living in sub-Saharan Africa.[1]

—THE REACH TRIAL[1]

Research Question(s): Would the use of hydroxyurea be effective in sub-Saharan African children with sickle cell disease (as compared with other regions of the world where its efficacy is established) despite concerns related to potential side effects or interactions with endemic diseases (like malaria) or comorbidities (like malnutrition)?

Funding: National Heart, Lung, and Blood Institute along with "others." Hydroxyurea was donated by the pharmaceutical company Bristol-Myers Squibb.

Year Study Began: Not indicated

Year Study Published: 2019

Study Location: Four countries in sub-Saharan Africa (Angola, Democratic Republic of Congo, Kenya, Uganda)

Who Was Studied: Children age 1–10 years

Who Was Excluded: Children <1 year old or >10 years old; children whose parents or guardians did not provide consent.

How Many Patients: 635

Study Overview: This study occurred in 3 distinct phases to allow for assessment of safety, feasibility, and efficacy of the intervention. First, there was a 2-month screening period to collect baseline, pre-treatment data. Second, participants received 6 months of the starting dose of hydroxyurea. Only after completing this second phase could participants enter the third phase of dose up-titration (see Figure 36.1).

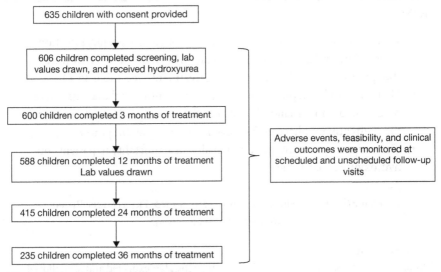

Figure 36.1. Overview of the study design.

Study Intervention: Provision of weight-based hydroxyurea doses in a dose-escalating fashion. The initial goal dose was 15–20 mg/kg/day (actual: 17.5 mg ± 1.8 mg/kg/day) for the first 6 months. Thereafter, the mean maximum tolerated dose was 22.5 ± 4.9 mg/kg/day. Lab values were drawn at baseline and 12 months after enrollment. Adverse events, feasibility, and clinical outcomes were monitored at both scheduled and unscheduled follow-up visits.

Follow-Up: 36 months

Endpoints:
Primary outcomes:
- Safety endpoints: Hematologic dose-limiting toxic effects in the first 3 months of hydroxyurea treatment in the first 133 children enrolled at each clinical trial site including:

- Hemoglobin <4.0 g/dL
- Absolute neutrophil count <1,000/mm^3
- Absolute reticulocyte count <80,000/mm^3 (if hemoglobin >7.0 g/dL)
- Platelet count <80,000/mm^3

Secondary outcomes:
- Feasibility (enrollment, retention, and adherence)
- Other safety endpoints
- Clinical benefits

RESULTS

- Hydroxyurea treatment reduced the rates of painful events, infection, transfusion, and death, with no increase in adverse events that were thought to be related to hydroxyurea treatment (see Table 36.1).
- Hydroxyurea had a protective effect on preventing malaria with a rate reduction of more than 50% (rate of 46.9 events per 100 patient years in the pretreatment phase vs. 22.9 events per 100 patient years).
- There was a significant reduction in all-cause mortality in patients on hydroxyurea (see Table 36.1).

Table 36.1 COMPARISON OF SCREENING AND TREATMENT PHASE
OUTCOMES, RESPECTIVELY

Adverse Events

Primary safety endpoint	5.1% (less than the 20% expected and 30% allowable)

Lab Values (after 1 year of hydroxyurea treatment)

Hemoglobin level	Increase of 1.0 g/dL (95% CI 0.8–1.0)
Mean Corpuscular volume	Increase of 13 fl (95% CI 12–13)
Fetal Hemoglobin Level	Increase of 12.5% (95% CI 11.8–13.1)

Clinical Benefits (selected)

Incidence all clinical adverse events	308.4 vs. 170.7/100 patient years Incidence rate ratio (IRR): 0.54 (95% CI 0.48–0.62)
Sickle cell–related events	114.5 vs. 53.0/100 patient years IRR: 0.47 (95% CI 0.38–0.57)
Non-malaria infection	142.5 vs. 90.0/100 patient years IRR: 0.62 (95% CI 0.53–0.72)
Malaria infection	46.9 vs. 22.9/100 patient years IRR: 0.49 (95% CI 0.37–0.66)
Blood transfusion	43.3 vs. 14.2/100 patient years IRR: 0.33 (95% CI 0.23–0.47)
Death	3.6 vs. 1.1/100 patient years IRR: 0.30 (95% CI 0.10–0.88)

Criticisms and Limitations:

- Since this was not a randomized trial, confounding factors may have biased the study results.
- This study forces us to ask hard ethical questions about whether and when well-established data (from higher-resource settings) need to be reproduced (at a high cost) in lower-resource settings to justify the use of known, effective medications/interventions in said lower-resource settings. Can the data from this study justify the use of hydroxyurea in South Asia, or do those nations need to produce their own trials? This is a tricky, gray area that can be argued from either perspective.

Other Relevant Studies and Information:

- Hydroxyurea is a myelosuppressive agent that raises the level of HbF in red blood cells and is well known to significantly reduce the frequency of sickle cell crises and chronic organ damage, and to prolong survival. It is on the World Health Organization (WHO) list of essential medicines for the treatment of hemoglobinopathies and is recommended for use in multiple other settings.[2]
- The REACH Trial's findings regarding malaria infection (while on hydroxyurea) extended previous findings from a study[3] (NOHARM) in Kampala, Uganda, which showed malaria infection rates were not higher on hydroxyurea as compared to placebo.
- Since the REACH Trial's completion, a similar study[4] in sub-Saharan African children demonstrated the superior clinical efficacy of dose escalation as compared to fixed-dose hydroxyurea with no differences in safety endpoints.

Summary and Implications: In lower-resource settings with the ability to perform follow-up and basic lab testing, hydroxyurea is feasible, safe, and effective among young children with sickle cell disease. Access to hydroxyurea should not be restricted due to concerns related to higher rates of certain infections (malaria) or comorbidities (malnutrition).

CLINICAL CASE: HYDROXYUREA FOR SICKLE CELL DISEASE

Case History

A mother brings her 5-year-old son and 3-year-old daughter to a clinic in rural Angola. Both children are known to have sickle cell disease (as did their late father). Neither child is on any form of treatment, but the 5-year-old has been admitted to the regional hospital 6 times in the past year for sickle cell–related complications or severe malaria infection. To date, the 3-year-old has been healthy. The mother reports that funds are very limited in their home due to the loss of her husband and these previous hospital admissions. She wonders what if anything can be done to help her son and worries about similar events occurring in the future for her daughter.

Suggested Answer

Assuming your rural clinic can perform some basic lab tests (complete blood count/hemogram, malaria smear or polymerase chain reaction [PCR]), it would be best to start both children on weight-based hydroxyurea with close follow-up to (1) monitor for adverse events and (2) plan dose up-titration. In the setting of their profound poverty, any government or social support system that can provide an essential medication like hydroxyurea to her at no (or minimal) cost would likely greatly aid in adherence.

References

1. Tshilolo L, Tomlinson G, Williams TN, et al. Hydroxyurea for children with sickle cell anemia in sub-Saharan Africa. *New Engl J Med*. 2018;380:121–131.
2. World Health Organization Model List of Essential Medicines, 21st List, 2019. Geneva: World Health Organization; 2019. Licence: CC BY-NC-SA 3.0 IGO.
3. Opoka RO, Ndugwa CM, Latham TS, et al. Novel use of hydroxyurea in an African region with malaria (NOHARM): A trial for children with sickle cell anemia. *Blood*. 2017;130:2585–2593.
4. John CC, Opoka RO, Latham TS, et al. Hydroxyurea dose escalation for sickle cell anemia in sub-Saharan Africa. *N Engl J Med*. 2020;382:2524–2533.

Women's Health

Our study selection in Section 5, Women's Health, mirrors the skew of research in resource-denied settings toward obstetrical issues rather than gynecologic issues. Four of the five chapters in this section are associated with maternal health, including aspirin in pregnancy for the prevention of preeclampsia, magnesium sulfate for the prevention of seizures in preeclampsia, tranexamic acid to treat postpartum hemorrhage, and the use of partograms in labor rooms to enable early and effective labor intervention. Visual inspection with acetic acid for cervical cancer screening was included, as this is often utilized in resource-denied settings instead of pap smear or HPV (human papillomavirus) testing to screen for a leading cause of cancer death in women globally that can be cured early with effective screening and treatment methods. There is some overlap with other sections again here, as we include a study on syndromic management of STDs in the infectious disease section. Notably absent is breast cancer screening, heavy menstrual bleeding, contraception, HPV vaccination, and abortion care. This is largely due to a paucity of studies applicable in low-resource settings or a lack of translation of research into practice.

SECTION

Women's Health

37

Does Prenatal Aspirin Prevent Preterm Preeclampsia?

Aspirin versus Placebo in Pregnancies at High Risk for Preterm Preeclampsia

MARIA OPENSHAW

The Combined Multimarker Screening and Randomized Patient Treatment with Aspirin for Evidence-Based Preeclampsia Prevention (ASPRE) Trial

This randomized trial showed that among women with singleton pregnancies who were identified by means of first-trimester screening as being at high risk for preterm preeclampsia, the administration of aspirin at a dose of 150 mg per day from 11 to 14 weeks of gestation until 36 weeks of gestation resulted in a significantly lower risk of preterm preeclampsia than with placebo.

—ROLNIK ET AL.[1]

Research Question: Does administration of low-dose aspirin in pregnant people at high risk of preeclampsia reduce the risk of preterm preeclampsia?

Funding: The European Union Seventh Framework Program and the Fetal Medicine Foundation

Year Study Began: 2014

Year Study Published: 2017

Study Location: 13 hospitals in the United Kingdom, Spain, Italy, Belgium, Greece, and Israel

Who Was Studied: Pregnant people at least 18 years of age; live, singleton pregnancy; high risk for preterm preeclampsia according to a screening algorithm that accounted for both demographic factors, history, and biomarkers.

Who Was Excluded: Unable to consent to participation (severely ill or unconscious; learning difficulties or serious mental illness); major fetal abnormality; known bleeding disorder; already taking aspirin or NSAID.

How Many Patients: 1776.

Study Overview: See Figure 37.1.

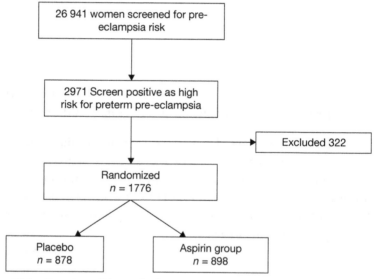

Figure 37.1. Overview of the study design.

Study Intervention: Pregnant people at high risk for preeclampsia were identified using a multimodal screening algorithm, a version of which is available at fetalmedicine.org/preeclampsia. Participants found to have high risk of preterm preeclampsia at 11–14 weeks by ultrasound dating were randomly assigned to receive either 150 mg of oral aspirin or placebo (tablets were identical). Participants were instructed to take one tablet every night throughout the trial until 36 weeks gestation or at the onset of labor, if occurring before 36 weeks.

Follow-Up: Adherence and adverse events were assessed at 3 follow-up clinical visits (19–24 weeks, 32–34 weeks, and 36 weeks); three telephone interviews (16 weeks, 28 weeks, and 30 days after completion of therapy). Clinical outcomes were assessed after delivery completion.

Endpoints: The primary outcome measure was delivery complicated by preeclampsia prior to 37 weeks gestation. Secondary outcomes included adverse outcomes before 34 weeks, before 37 weeks, and at or after 37 weeks; stillbirth or neonatal death; neonatal complications, neonatal therapy and poor fetal growth.

RESULTS

- Preterm preeclampsia occurred in 13/798 participants (1.6%) in the aspirin group, compared to 35/822 (4.3%) in the placebo group. Participants who received aspirin were 62% less likely to have preterm preeclampsia (AOR 0.38; 95% CI 0.20–0.74, $p = 0.004$).
- The effect size was consistent across estimated risk groups, relative to obstetric history, and across countries of participating centers.
- There was no significant difference in the incidence of any secondary outcome (e.g., preeclampsia, gestational hypertension, small-for-gestational age, miscarriage/stillbirth, abruption, or spontaneous preterm delivery; stillbirth, low birthweight, NICU admission, death or serious neonatal complication); however, the study was insufficiently powered to detect these differences.
- There was no difference in the number of serious adverse events (1.6% in aspirin group versus 3.2% in placebo) or adverse events (25.9% in aspirin group and 25.5% in placebo) (Table 37.1).
- Adherence was good in 79.9% of participants, moderate in 14.9%, and poor in 5.2%; there were no significant between-group differences in the level of adherence.

Table 37.1 SELECT KEY FINDINGS: MATERNAL AND NEONATAL OUTCOMES
ACCORDING TO TRIAL GROUP

Outcome	Aspirin Group (n = 798)	Placebo Group (n = 822)	Odds Ratio
Preterm preeclampsia at <37 weeks gestation *(Primary outcome)*	13 (1.6%)	35 (4.3%)	0.38 (0.20–0.74)
Any adverse outcome at <34 weeks gestation	32 (4.0%)	53 (6.4%)	0.62 (0.34–1.14)
Any adverse outcome at <37 weeks gestation	79 (9.9%)	116 (14.1%)	0.69 (0.46–1.03)
Any adverse outcome at ≥37 weeks gestation	178 (22.3%)	171 (20.8%)	1.12 (0.82–1.54)
Any stillbirth or death	8 (1.0%)	14 (1.7%)	0.59 (0.19–1.85)
Any death or complication	32 (4.0%)	48 (5.8%)	0.69 (0.37–1.27)
Admission to neonatal intensive care unit	48 (6.0%)	54 (6.6%)	0.93 (0.55–1.59)
Poor fetal growth <5%ile *(birth weights <24 weeks were not recorded)*	82/785 (7.3%)	96/807 (11.9%)	0.86 (0.57–1.30)

Criticisms and Limitations:

While the study's innovative "combined multimarker screening" for women at high risk of preterm preeclampsia (which included demographic characteristics, historical factors, and biomarkers including serum screening and uterine artery ultrasound) yielded a greater impact on the target outcome, this approach is impractical in middle- or low-resource settings where targeted screening is unavailable. While low-dose aspirin is touted as a low-cost intervention, study staff conducted blood work and specialized ultrasound screening for 26 941 women while preventing an estimated 22 cases of preterm preeclampsia in the intervention group.

Other Relevant Studies and Information:

- Most obstetric guidelines recommend administration of low-dose aspirin to women at high risk of preeclampsia, but there is no consensus definition of "high risk."[2–4]
- A 2007 meta-analysis of 31 randomized controlled trials (RCTs) suggested that antiplatelet agents such as low-dose aspirin are safe and effective in reducing preeclampsia and associated adverse events, but

with large numbers needed to treat (143 to prevent a delivery prior to 34 weeks and 333 to prevent a perinatal death).[5,6]

- Similarly, a 2014 meta-analysis found a pooled 24% reduction in preeclampsia with the use of low-dose aspirin, but noted heterogeneity in screening criteria used to determine high-risk status, with control group preeclampsia rates ranging from 8% to 30%.[7] However, there was no significant effect on perinatal mortality.
- Since the effect size of the intervention varies based on preeclampsia rates in the target population, researchers have sought to improve the algorithm for preeclampsia risk. By incorporating maternal and placental biomarkers into the algorithm, the Fetal Medicine Foundation algorithm has improved sensitivity, detecting 100% (95% CI 80%–100%) of preeclampsia <32 weeks, 75% (95% CI 62%–85%) of preeclampsia <37 weeks and 43% (95% CI 35%–50%) of preeclampsia ≥37 weeks, with a 10.0% false positive rate.[8]

Summary and Implications: This study found that universal screening among pregnant people for risk of preeclampsia can effectively identify those at high risk who would benefit from treatment with low-dose aspirin (75–150 mg) starting between 11 and 14 weeks gestation. Perinatal care providers should use the best available evidence to determine preeclampsia risk; in most settings, this consists of a review of historical and demographic factors; in high-resource settings, biometric screening factors including uterine artery ultrasound can be incorporated for improved sensitivity when available. Regardless of whether an individual chooses to take low-dose aspirin during pregnancy, all pregnant people should undergo routine blood pressure screening in pregnancy and education regarding the signs and symptoms of preeclampsia.

CLINICAL CASE: PREVENTING RECURRENT PREECLAMPSIA

Case History

You are a consultant with an NGO in Malawi. You have been asked to look at the formulary in the prenatal ward and suggest what medications should be stocked. There is a high rate of maternal death from preeclampsia in this region. What medicines would you recommend stocking in order to decrease maternal and neonatal morbidity and mortality from preeclampsia?

Suggested Answer

Medications that are recommended by the World Health Organization to prevent preeclampsia include low-dose aspirin and calcium (at doses of 1.5–2.0g elemental Ca/day) in patients with poor calcium intake.

For prevention and treatment of eclampsia, you should keep vials of IM or IV magnesium sulfate on hand. Severe range blood pressures (SBP $\geq$160, DBP $\geq$110) should be treated with anti-hypertensive medications such as nifedipine PO, IV labetalol, IV hydralazine, or methyldopa.

With breakdowns in supply chains occurring commonly for a variety of reasons, it can be difficult to maintain stocks of medicines. However, these medications can be lifesaving and help prevent and treat preeclampsia and eclampsia and therefore should be prioritized.

References

1. Rolnik DL, Wright D, Poon LC, et al. Aspirin versus placebo in pregnancies at high risk for preterm preeclampsia. *N Engl J Med.* 2017;377(7):613–622. doi: 10.1056/NEJMoa1704559

2. American College of Obstetricians and Gynecologists. Low-dose aspirin use during pregnancy. *ACOG Comm Opin Number* 743. 2018;132(1):e44–e52.

3. National Institute for Health and Care Excellent (NICE). Hypertension in pregnancy: Diagnosis and management. Published online June 25, 2019. https://www.nice.org.uk/guidance/ng133

4. Poon LC, Shennan A, Hyett JA, et al. The International Federation of Gynecology and Obstetrics (FIGO) initiative on pre-eclampsia: A pragmatic guide for first-trimester screening and prevention. *Int J Gynecol Obstet.* 2019;145(S1):1–33. doi: 10.1002/ijgo.12802

5. Askie LM, Duley L, Henderson-Smart DJ, Stewart LA. Antiplatelet agents for prevention of pre-eclampsia: A meta-analysis of individual patient data. *Lancet.* 2007;369(9575):1791–1798. doi: 10.1016/S0140-6736(07)60712-0

6. Greene MF, Solomon CG. Aspirin to prevent preeclampsia. *N Engl J Med.* 2017;377(7):690–691. doi:1 0.1056/NEJMe1708920

7. Henderson JT, Whitlock EP, O'Connor E, Senger CA, Thompson JH, Rowland MG. Low-dose aspirin for prevention of morbidity and mortality from preeclampsia: A systematic evidence review for the U.S. Preventive Services Task Force. *Ann Intern Med.* 2014;160(10):695–703. doi: 10.7326/M13-2844

8. O'Gorman N, Wright D, Poon LC, et al. Multicenter screening for pre-eclampsia by maternal factors and biomarkers at 11-13 weeks' gestation: Comparison with NICE guidelines and ACOG recommendations. *Ultrasound Obstet Gynecol.* 2017;49(6):756–760. doi: 10.1002/uog.17455

38

Can Tranexamic Acid Stop Postpartum Hemorrhage?

The WOMAN Trial

ALEXA LINDLEY, MARIANA MONTANO, AND ROSE L. MOLINA

Tranexamic acid reduces death due to bleeding in women with post-partum hemorrhage with no adverse effects. When used as a treatment for postpartum hemorrhage, tranexamic acid should be given as soon as possible after bleeding onset.[1]

—EFFECT OF EARLY TRANEXAMIC ACID ADMINISTRATION ON
MORTALITY, HYSTERECTOMY, AND OTHER MORBIDITIES IN WOMEN
WITH POST-PARTUM HAEMORRHAGE (WOMAN): AN INTERNATIONAL,
RANDOMISED, DOUBLE-BLIND, PLACEBO-CONTROLLED TRIAL
[PUBLISHED CORRECTION APPEARS IN LANCET. 2017 MAY
27;389(10084):2104]. LANCET. 2017;389(10084):2105–2116.
DOI:10.1016/S0140-6736(17)30638-4

Research Question: Does early administration of tranexamic acid prevent death, hysterectomy, and other relevant outcomes in women with postpartum hemorrhage?

Funding: London School of Hygiene & Tropical Medicine, Pfizer, UK Department of Health, Wellcome Trust, and Bill & Melinda Gates Foundation

Year Study Began: 2010

Year Study Ended: 2016

Year Study Published: 2017

Study Location: 193 hospitals in 21 countries

Who Was Studied: Women aged 16 years and older with a clinical diagnosis of postpartum hemorrhage after a vaginal birth or cesarean birth.

Who Was Excluded: Patients who had hysterectomy prior to randomization, those who withdrew consent after randomization.

How Many Patients Enrolled: 20 060

Study Overview: See Figure 38.1.

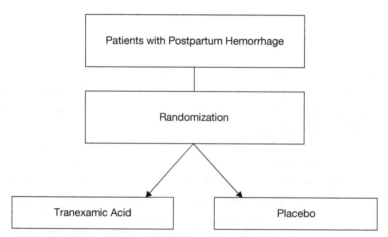

Figure 38.1. Overview of the study design.

Study Intervention: Patients diagnosed with postpartum hemorrhage by clinical criteria (defined as estimated blood loss of greater than 500 cc after vaginal birth, greater than 1000 cc after cesarean birth, or any bleeding sufficient to compromise hemodynamic instability) were randomized to receive either 1 g tranexamic acid or placebo by slow intravenous injection in addition to usual care. If bleeding continued after 30 minutes or recurred during the first 24 hours after the first dose, a second dose of either tranexamic acid or placebo was administered.

Follow-Up: Outcomes were collected until death, discharge from hospital, or 42 days after randomization if still in the hospital (whichever happened first).

Endpoints:

Primary outcome: composite of death from all causes or hysterectomy.

Secondary outcomes: death due to bleeding, thromboembolic events, surgical interventions, complications, adverse events, quality of life, and thromboembolic events in breastfed newborns.

RESULTS

- There was no difference in the primary endpoint of all-cause mortality or hysterectomy for patients receiving tranexamic acid (occurred in 5.3%) compared to patients receiving placebo (occurred in 5.6%), 95% CI 0.87–1.09, $p = 0.65$ (Table 38.1).
- There was a statistically significant decrease in death due to hemorrhage for patients who received tranexamic acid (1.5%) compared to the placebo (1.9%, 95% CI 0.65–1.00, $p = 0.045$, number needed to treat [NNT] 250).
- In a subgroup analysis, patients who were treated with tranexamic acid within 3 hours of delivery had a statistically significant decrease in risk of death due to bleeding compared to those in the placebo group (1.2% vs. 1.7%, respectively, 95% CI 0.52–0.91, $p = 0.008$). There was no difference in death from bleeding when tranexamic acid or placebo was given later than 3 hours after delivery (2.6% vs. 2.5%, respectively, 95% CI 0.76–1.51, $p = 0.70$).
- There were no statistically significant differences in the thromboembolic events, complications, adverse events, quality of life, or thromboembolic events in breastfed newborns in the tranexamic acid group compared to placebo group.

Table 38.1 SUMMARY OF THE STUDY'S KEY FINDINGS

Outcome	Tranexamic Acid Group	Placebo Group	p Value
All-cause mortality or hysterectomy	5.3%	5.6%	0.65
Death due to postpartum hemorrhage	1.5%	1.9%	0.045

Criticisms and Limitations:

- The study hypothesis was refined and the sample size was increased after the study was underway because the decision to proceed with hysterectomy often coincided with the decision for enrollment in the trial, which may have diminished the effect of tranexamic acid on the risk of hysterectomy.
- Injectable tranexamic acid may be unfeasible to use in some resource-limited settings due to cost or availability.
- Reduction in cause-specific mortality narrowly reached statistical significance in the tranexamic acid group, and concerns about ascertainment of cause of death may limit the strength of the conclusions.

Other Relevant Studies:

- A trial evaluating prophylactic tranexamic acid administration in women with vaginal delivery did not demonstrate a decreased incidence of postpartum hemorrhage compared to placebo.[2]
- A systematic review and meta-analysis evaluating prophylactic tranexamic acid administration for women undergoing cesarean delivery found that tranexamic acid reduces postpartum hemorrhage and need for red blood cell transfusion.[3]
- The World Health Organization recommends the administration of tranexamic acid within 3 hours of birth for any patient clinically diagnosed with postpartum hemorrhage following vaginal birth or caesarean delivery.[4]

Summary and Implications: Although this trial found that tranexamic acid does not decrease all-cause mortality or hysterectomy, it did show a statistically significant decrease in death from postpartum hemorrhage. With a number needed to treat of 250, the effect is modest. However, given that there were no complications associated with tranexamic acid treatment, this trial supports its use in the treatment of postpartum hemorrhage, which is the leading cause of maternal mortality worldwide.

CLINICAL CASE: MANAGEMENT OF POSTPARTUM HEMORRHAGE

Case History
A 30-year-old gravida 3, para 2 at 39 weeks and 5 days gestation presents to Labor and Delivery with regular uterine contractions. Initial vital signs are normal and a sterile vaginal exam reveals 5 cm of cervical dilation, 80% effacement, and –1 station. Labor progresses spontaneously and she delivers a vigorous infant vaginally without complications. Active management of the third stage is performed. After delivery of the placenta, rapid vaginal bleeding begins and quickly reaches an estimated blood loss of 800 cc. Uterine palpation reveals poor uterine tone. A postpartum hemorrhage protocol is started, including administration of uterotonic medications.

Based on the results of the WOMAN trial, would you administer IV tranexamic acid for this patient? If so, at what point in the protocol would you order it?

Suggested Answer
According to the WOMAN trial, administration of IV tranexamic acid, in addition to usual postpartum hemorrhage management, decreases maternal death due to postpartum hemorrhage. This effect was only present if tranexamic acid was given within 3 hours of delivery, so if given, tranexamic acid should be administered soon after delivery. In this case it would be reasonable to treat this patient with tranexamic acid along with routine postpartum hemorrhage care.

References

1. WOMAN Trial Collaborators. Effect of early tranexamic acid administration on mortality, hysterectomy, and other morbidities in women with post-partum haemorrhage (WOMAN): An international, randomised, double-blind, placebo-controlled trial [published correction appears in Lancet. 2017 May 27;389(10084):2104]. *Lancet.* 2017;389(10084):2105–2116. doi: 10.1016/S0140-6736(17)30638-4
2. Sentilhes L, Winer N, Azria E, et al. Tranexamic acid for the prevention of blood loss after vaginal delivery. *N Engl J Med.* 2018;379(8):731–742. doi: 10.1056/NEJMoa1800942
3. Franchini M, Mengoli C, Cruciani M, et al. Safety and efficacy of tranexamic acid for prevention of obstetric haemorrhage: An updated systematic review and meta-analysis. *Blood Transfus.* 2018;16(4):329–337. doi: 10.2450/2018.0026-18
4. World Health Organization. WHO recommendation on tranexamic acid for the treatment of postpartum haemorrhage. *Lancet.* 2017;389(10084):2105–2116. doi: 10.1016/S0140-6736(17)30638-4

39

Magnesium Sulphate for Seizure Prophylaxis in Women with Preeclampsia

The Magpie Trial

ANDREA WALKER

> Magnesium sulphate halves the risk of eclampsia, and probably reduces the risk of maternal death. There do not appear to be substantive harmful effects to mother or baby in the short term.
> —THE MAGNESIUM SULPHATE FOR PREVENTION OF ECLAMPSIA
> (MAGPIE) TRIAL COLLABORATIVE GROUP[1]

Research Question: Do women with preeclampsia and their babies benefit from magnesium sulphate?[1]

Funding: UK Medical Research Council, UK Department for International Development, UNDP/UNFPA/WHO/World Bank Special Programme of Research, Development and Research Training in Human Reproduction

Year Study Began: 1998

Year Study Published: 2002

Study Location: 33 countries

Who Was Studied: Pregnant women with singleton or multiple gestations with preeclampsia (blood pressure >140 mmHg systolic and/or >90 mmHg diastolic on 2 separate occasions with documented proteinuria) who had not yet delivered or were less than 24 hours postpartum.

Who Was Excluded: Patients with a known hypersensitivity to magnesium, history of myasthenia gravis, or those in a hepatic coma at risk of renal failure were excluded.

How Many Patients: 10 141

Study Overview:

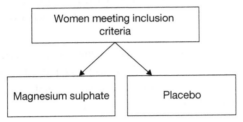

Figure 39.1. Summary of Magpie Trial Design.

Study Intervention: Patients were randomized to receive a 4 g loading dose of either magnesium sulphate (MgSO4) or placebo, followed by 24 hours of maintenance therapy which was either administered intramuscular (IM) or intravenous (IV). The IV maintenance dosing was 1 g/hour, while the IM dosing included 10 g IM in combination with the initial IV loading dose, followed by 5 g IM q4 hours.

Magnesium toxicity was evaluated by serial reflex exams every 30 minutes and urine output monitored hourly. Magnesium dosing was reduced by half when there was evidence of toxicity or low urine output. If a patient had an eclamptic seizure the trial treatment was stopped and non-trial magnesium sulphate was started.

Follow-Up: Until discharge from the hospital

Endpoints: Primary outcomes: eclampsia, fetal death. Secondary outcomes: significant maternal morbidity (as individual, pre-specified outcomes and as a composite), complications of labor including cesarean section, and neonatal morbidity.

RESULTS

- In the MgSO4 group, there was a 58% risk reduction of eclampsia when compared to the placebo arm. The number needed to treat to prevent an eclamptic seizure in women with severe preeclampsia was 63, and was 109 for mild preeclampsia.

- There was no difference in the risk of maternal death between the two groups (RR 0.55, 95% CI 0.26–1.14). MgSO4 did not affect maternal morbidity compared to the placebo when evaluating for respiratory depression, respiratory arrest, pulmonary edema, cardiac arrest, renal failure, or liver failure.
- There was a lower risk of placental abruption in patients who received MgSO4 prior to delivery. The article cites 12 fewer placental abruptions per 1000 women.
- Women who received MgSO4 during the labor process were noted to have a 5% higher risk of requiring a cesarean section (RR 1.05%, CI 1.00–1.11, $p = 0.02$).
- There was no difference in length of hospital stay or need for admission to an intensive care unit between the placebo and MgSO4 groups.
- There was no difference in the in-utero or neonatal death rate between the two groups (RR 1.02, 95% CI 0.92–1.14).
- There was no difference in effectiveness of MgSO4 when comparing intramuscular versus intravenous routes of administration.

Criticisms and Limitations: The most important limitation of this study is the evolving definition of preeclampsia with and without severe features. The Magpie Study utilizes a classic definition of preeclampsia. Blood pressure parameters and definitions of proteinuria have changed slightly since then, as have qualifying laboratory and clinical characteristics that classify a patient as severe. Despite these newer definitions, the benefits of magnesium remain steadfast and the therapy is still considered first-line treatment in the prevention of eclampsia in women with preeclampsia.

Although the Magpie Trial is a large, multicenter, randomized controlled trial, the MgSO4 arm had a significantly higher rate of maternal side effects such as hot flashes and nausea. Therefore, the presence of these side effects could have inadvertently unblinded the study. It is estimated that approximately 20% of the women allocated MgSO4 were able to determine which treatment they were receiving. The clinical significance of this remains unknown.

The study did not randomize route of administration for magnesium; therefore, the assumptions made about equipoise between IM and IV routes of magnesium should be considered with caution; however, both routes were used and it is reasonable to consider the IM route in resource-denied areas or in clinical scenarios where intravenous access is not available.

Other Relevant Studies and Information:

- A follow-up study by the Magpie Collaborative Group evaluated long-term maternal and neonatal effects 2 years after receiving MgSO4. There was no increase in the risk of death or disability.[2] Despite the clear advantages of magnesium sulfate in preventing maternal morbidity from preeclampsia, many barriers to its use exist in low- and middle-income countries (LMIC) such as: unreliable supply of the medicine and the materials required for its administration, lack of training of healthcare providers about MgSO4 administration, and lack of political will to change procurement of and licensing protocols for MgSO4.
- These findings have also been validated in LMIC; however, due to concerns over magnesium toxicity, alternative (lower) dosing regimens are typically used, including loading dose only regimens, though the lowest effective dosing regimen remains unclear.[3]
- Through task shifting, community administration of a MgSO4 loading dose before transfer to a health facility was associated with a lower rate of eclampsia recurrence (RR 0.23, 95% CI 0.11–0.49) than transfer and MgSO4 administration in the care facility.[4]
- The MAGPIE study demonstrated that MgSO4 reduces eclamptic seizure in patients with mild preeclampsia. However, subsequent reviews of available trials do not demonstrate a clear improvement in maternal or fetal outcomes in this cohort;[5] thus, WHO guidelines do not currently recommend the universal use of magnesium sulfate in preeclampsia without severe features.[6]

Summary and Implications: Magnesium sulphate therapy reduces the risk of eclampsia by 58% without increasing maternal or fetal morbidity from the treatment.

CLINICAL CASE: MAGNESIUM SULPHATE THERAPY FOR SEIZURE PROPHYLAXIS

Case History

After a maternal and neonatal death due to eclampsia at a rural health clinic, the Ministry of Health asks you to write up a list of supplies and strategies that a rural health clinic may need to help prevent future events such as this. Based on the findings of the Magpie Trial and other studies in this book, what sorts of interventions might you recommend putting in place?

Suggested Answer

The Magpie Trial demonstrated a reduced risk of eclamptic convulsions with magnesium sulphate. There is no difference in the efficacy of IM magnesium sulphate versus IV administration, and IM administration is often easier to provide in resource-denied settings. Sufficient stock of intramuscular magnesium as well as the required materials for administration (syringes, needles, alcohol swabs) should be readily available for emergencies such as this. If not already, magnesium sulfate should be added to the country's essential medication list, as well as calcium gluconate for managing toxicity.

In addition to initiating magnesium sulphate, prompt anti-hypertensive therapy should be initiated in this scenario, and appropriate medications should be available.

To help prevent the development of preeclampsia in women receiving prenatal care at the clinic, the World Health Organization (WHO) recommends routine calcium supplementation in areas with low calcium intake, as well as daily low-dose aspirin administration for women at high risk of developing preeclampsia.[6]

Ensuring political support, adequate stock, clear guidelines for administration of these medications, and educating personnel on these guidelines may help prevent these outcomes.

References

1. Duley L, Magpie Trial Collaboration Group. Do women with pre-eclampsia, and their babies, benefit from magnesium sulphate? The Magpie Trial: A randomized placebo-controlled trial. *Lancet.* 2002; 359:1877–1890.
2. Magpie Trial Follow-Up Study Collaborative Group. The Magpie Trial: A randomized trial comparing magnesium sulphate with placebo for pre-eclampsia. Outcome for women at 2 years. *BJOG.* 2007;114:300–309.
3. Gordon R, Magee LA, Payne B, et al. Magnesium sulphate for the management of preeclampsia and eclampsia in low and middle income countries: A systematic review of tested dosing regimens. *J Obstet Gynaecol Can.* 2014 Feb;36(2):154–163. doi: 10.1016/S1701-2163(15)30662-9. PMID: 24518915.
4. Shamsuddin L, Nahar K, Nasrin B, et al. Use of parenteral magnesium sulphate in eclampsia and severe pre-eclampsia cases in a rural set up of Bangladesh. *Bangladesh Med Res Counc Bull.* 2005;31:75–82.
5. Sibai BM. Magnesium sulfate prophylaxis in preeclampsia: Lessons learned from recent trials. *Am J Obstet Gynecol.* 2004 Jun;190(6):1520–1526. Review. PubMed PMID: 15284724.
6. *WHO Recommendations for Prevention and Treatment of Pre-Eclampsia and Eclampsia.* Geneva: World Health Organization Press; 2011.

40

Effects of Partograms on Birthing Outcomes in Developing Nations

NAKYDA DEAN

[M]onitoring labour with a partogram allows early detection of fetal distress (with the alert line) and of stillbirth (with the action line).... [T]hese results show the usefulness and efficacy of the partogram and underscore the value of medical intervention as soon as the alert line is crossed.

—DUJARDIN ET AL.[1]

Research Question: How do the alert line and action line on the partogram affect birth outcomes in developing nations?

Funding: None declared

Year Study Began: 1990

Year Study Published: 1992

Study Location: 4 maternity clinics in Pikine, Senegal

Who Was Studied: All pregnant patients who presented to 4 peripheral maternity clinics whose labor was monitored with a partogram.

Who Was Excluded: About 20% of the pregnant population, who opted for a home delivery, were excluded from the study. Other pregnant patients were excluded from the study if partograms were not available due to an unexpected delivery at home or en route, emergency transfer on admission, or complete dilation on admission.

How Many Patients: 1022

Study Overview: Prospective multicenter observational study (see Figure 40.1).

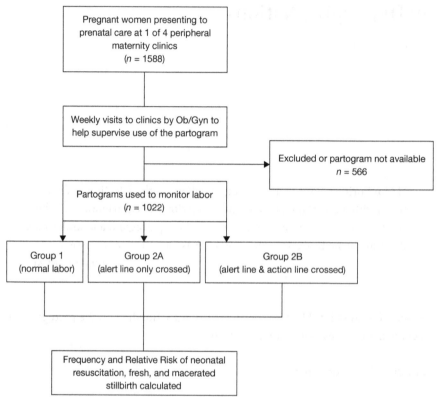

Figure 40.1. Overview of the study design.

Study Intervention: A partogram is a low-tech paper graph that can be utilized to monitor a patient's labor progress (see Figure 40.2). It contains two diagonal lines labeled "Alert" and "Action" that indicate a slowly progressing labor and the need for intervention (transfer to another facility, augmentation of labor, cesarean section) if the labor is not progressing normally. In this study, all laboring women had partograms filled out by staff with maternal health information, the woman's labor progress, documentation of any medical management of labor dystocia if it occurred, and neonatal outcomes. An obstetrician/gynecologist visited every week during the length of the study to supervise and review the documentation.

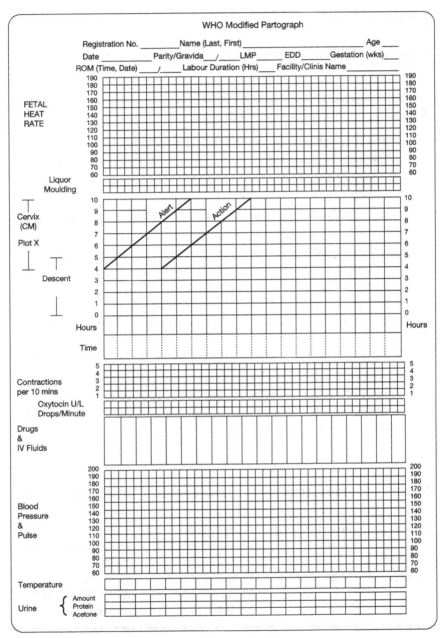

Figure 40.2. Modified WHO partograph, reproduced.

The labor was categorized into two main categories: (1) normal labor and (2) abnormal labor. The second group was divided into two subgroups: (i) alert line crossed and (ii) alert line and action line crossed. The outcomes were then compared between the groups.

Follow-Up: None

Endpoints: Frequency of neonatal resuscitation and stillborn rates

RESULTS

- Of the 1022 patients, the alert line was crossed in 100 (9.8%) cases. The action line was crossed in 35 of all cases (3.4%), which represented 35% of all cases crossing the alert line.
- For labors that crossed the alert line, neonatal resuscitation was 4 times more likely than for the normal labor group (RR 4.0, 95% CI 2.3–7.1; $p <$ 0.0001).
- For labors that crossed the alert line and the action line, the relative risk for fresh stillbirth was approximately 10-fold in comparison to normal labor (RR 9.9, 95% CI 2.8–34.7; $p < 0.001$).
- Crossing the alert line has a sensitivity of 27%, a specificity of 93%, and a positive predictive value of 17% for the neonate needing resuscitation at birth.
- Augmentation of labor (artificial rupture of membrane, administration of oxytocin) took place in half of the cases with abnormal labor. For patients who received treatment, only 26% of cases reached the action line, compared to 44% crossing the action line when intervention did not take place ($p = 0.06$) (Table 40.1).

Table 40.1 SUMMARY OF KEY FINDINGS

Outcome	Normal Labor	Alert Line Crossed (RR)	Alert and Action Lines Crossed (RR)
Resuscitation	4.3% (38/880)	17.2% (10/58) RR 4.0 (CI 2.3–7.1) $p <0.01$	17.4 (4/23) RR 4.0 (CI 1.6–10.3) $p = 0.02$
Stillbirths	2.2% (21/919)	7.3% (7/95) RR 3.2 (CI 1.4–7.4) $p <0.05$	9.7% (3/31) RR 9.9 (CI 2.8–34.7) $p <0.001$

Criticisms and Limitations:

- The partogram used in this study is an older version and varies from the modified WHO model (Figure 40.2).

- There is no clear consensus on the definitions or time frames of "normal labor," and the alert and action lines are based on labor data from the 1950s which may not be applicable to a wide range of populations or contemporary women.
- This partogram is not self-explanatory, requires training on how to use it, and can be cumbersome. There is wide variation in use among hospitals and even providers within hospitals in the appropriate completion and use of the partogram.[2] Studies have shown under-utilization of this tool, with complete use averaging 40%–60%.[3,4]
- Although the partogram may result in recognition and treatment of prolonged labor, deficiencies in staffing, supplies, and availability of further maternity care may limit its efficacy in improving outcomes.[5]

Other Relevant Studies and Information:

- Approximately 800 women die from preventable causes related to pregnancy and childbirth daily, and 99% of all maternal deaths occur in developing countries.[6]
- Detection of prolonged labor is important, as this is associated with increased maternal and neonatal morbidity such as postpartum hemorrhage, infection, and fistula formation. These risks are greater in low-income countries with resource limitations.
- The partograph has been called one of the most important advances in modern obstetric care and is recommended by WHO in monitoring the first stage of labor and therefore preventing prolonged or obstructive labor and maternal deaths.
- The data supporting the use of partograms for improving outcomes are conflicting. A Cochrane review showed that using the partogram as part of routine care is not associated with improvements in outcomes.[7] However, the trials included in the review were mainly conducted in high-income countries where there are significant concerns regarding over-intervention. On the other hand, data from resource-limited settings have shown that using the modified WHO partograph appears to improve outcomes including reduced caesarean section rate, augmentation of labor, perinatal outcomes, and timely transfers.[2,8–10]

Summary and Implications: This study based in a resource-limited setting found that an abnormal partogram is associated with fetal distress. Crossing the alert line is associated with increased relative risk for neonatal resuscitation and stillbirth. When the alert line is crossed, this should be an indication to augment labor and/or transfer to a higher level of care, and for staff to be ready for possible need for neonatal resuscitation at birth. However, for this to be effective, the patient's labor must be monitored, the partogram must be filled out accurately and followed accurately, and interventions and/or ability to transfer must be readily available.

CLINICAL CASE: PARTOGRAM

Case History

A 26-year-old G3P2 at 38w6d has been admitted to the maternity ward for labor at a local health clinic with no operative capabilities. On admission at 1900, she was 6 cm dilated, with 4/5 descent, having 3 moderate strength contractions every 10 minutes with normal fetal heart tones. Two hours later she was checked and was 8 cm dilated with 3/5 descent with 3 moderate strength contractions every 10 minutes. Shortly after, she had spontaneous rupture of membranes with clear fluid. At 2300 vaginal exam was still 8 cm dilated, with 4/5 descent, and 3 moderate contractions every 10 minutes.

Based on the WHO modified partogram (see Figure 40.2) and the information from this study, has the alert line been crossed, and what actions should be taken?

Suggested Answer

Using the WHO modified partogram, the labor progress was as expected from the first to the second vaginal check. However, with the third check the alert line was crossed, which represents protracted labor, and augmentation of labor is recommended. The patient may benefit from referral to a health center with ability for augmentation with oxytocin. The patient's partogram should be sent with the patient so that her labor can continue to be followed and plotted.

According to this study, crossing the alert line has a 4-fold increased risk for neonatal resuscitation. It may be prudent to be ready for neonatal resuscitation at birth. Monitoring the labor with the partogram can alert healthcare workers to start medical interventions when the labor progress is abnormal. This can decrease the proportion of women that cross the action line. Labors that cross the alert and action line have a relative risk of fresh stillbirths of approximately 10.

References

1. Dujardin B, De Schampheleire I, Sene H, Ndiaye F. Value of the alert and action lines on the partogram. *Lancet.* 1992 May 30;339:1336–1338.

2. Yisma E, Dessalegn B, Astatkie A, Fesseha N. Completion of the modified World Health Organization (WHO) partograph during labour in public health institutions of Addis Ababa, Ethiopia. *Reprod Health.* 2013;10:23. Published 2013 Apr 18. doi:10.1186/1742-4755-10-23

3. Opoku BK, Nguah SB. Utilization of the modified WHO partograph in assessing the progress of labour in a metropolitan area in Ghana. Research Journal of Women's Health. 2015;2(1):2. doi:https://doi.org/10.7243/2054-9865-2-2

4. Mukisa J, Grant I, Magala J, Ssemata AS, Lumala PZ, Byamugisha J. Level of partograph completion and healthcare workers' perspectives on its use in Mulago National Referral and teaching hospital, Kampala, Uganda. *BMC Health Serv Res.* 2019 Feb;19(1):107. doi: 10.1186/s12913-019-3934-3

5. Ollerhead E, Osrin D. Barriers to and incentives for achieving partograph use in obstetric practice in low- and middle-income countries: a systematic review. *BMC Pregnancy Childbirth.* 2014;14:281. Published 2014 Aug 16. doi: 10.1186/1471-2393-14-281

6. World Health Organization. *Preventing Prolonged Labour: A Practical Guide; The Partograph, Part I: Principles and Strategy, Part II: User's Manual, Part III: Facilitator's Manual, Part IV: Guidelines for Operations Research.* World Health Organization; 1994.

7. Bedwell C, Levin K, Pett C, Lavender DT. A realist review of the partograph: When and how does it work for labour monitoring? *BMC Pregnancy Childbirth.* 2017 Jan;17(1):31. doi: 10.1186/s12884-016-1213-4

8. Housseine N, Punt MC, Browne JL, et al. Strategies for intrapartum foetal surveillance in low- and middle-income countries: A systematic review. *PLoS ONE.* 2018;13(10): e0206295. https://doi.org/10.1371/journal.pone.0206295

9. Dalal AR, Purandare AC. The partograph in childbirth: An absolute essentiality or a mere exercise? *J Obstet Gynaecol India.* 2018;68(1):3–14. doi: 10.1007/s13224-017-1051-y

10. Lavender T, Omoni G, Lee K, et al. Student nurses experiences of using the partograph in labor wards in Kenya: A qualitative study. *Afr J Midwifery Womens Health.* 2011;5(3):117–122. doi: 10.12968/ajmw.2011.5.3.117

41

What Is a Cost-Effective Way to Screen for Cervical Cancer in Resource-Denied Settings?

STEPHANIE SIRNA

[Screening with visual inspection], in the presence of good training and sustained quality assurance, is an effective method to prevent cervical cancer in developing countries.

—SANKARANARAYANAN ET AL.[1]

Research Question: Does visual inspection with 4% acetic acid (vinegar [VIA]) impact cervical cancer incidence and mortality?

Funding: Bill & Melinda Gates Foundation through the Alliance for Cervical Cancer Prevention (ACCP), Seattle, USA

Years of Study: 1999/2000–2006; enumeration of households and eligible women started in October 1999, and screening began in January 2000.

Year of Publishing: 2007

Study Location: 114 municipal units (clusters) in 7 sub-districts of Dindigul district, Tamil Nadu, India

Who Was Studied: Women aged 30–59 years, apparently healthy, with intact uterus and no prior history of cervical cancer living in the above clusters.

Who was Excluded: Women with non-intact uterus or prior history of cervical cancer.

Number of patients: 80 282 total (49 311 intervention arm and 30 962 control arm)

Study Overview: See Figure 41.1.

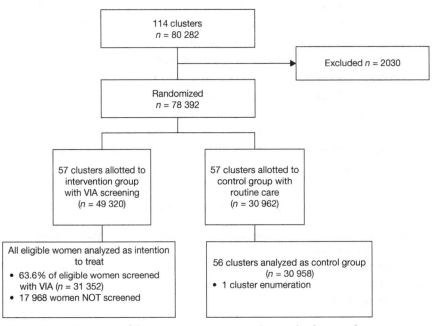

Figure 41.1. Overview of this intention-to-treat randomized cohort study.

Study Intervention: Patients in the intervention group were assigned to receive single round of VIA screening by a trained nurse plus routine care. The women in the control group received routine care, which consisted of promotion of preventive services and education regarding access to services, cancer screening education, signs and symptoms of cervical cancer, early detection, and treatment.

Follow-Up: 1, 3, 5 and 7 years

Endpoints:
  Primary outcome: cervical cancer incidence and mortality.
  Secondary outcome measures: FIGO (International Federation of Obstetrics and Gynecology) stage distribution.

RESULTS

- Overall, there was a 25% reduction in cervical cancer incidence rate in the intervention group, adjusted hazard ratio (HR) 0.75 (CI 0.59–0.95) (adjusted for age, education, marital status, parity, and cluster design); however, age-group analysis showed that this was only significant in the 30–39-year age group.
- There was an overall 35% reduction in cervical cancer mortality in the intervention group compared to the control group, adjusted HR 0.65 (CI 0.47–0.89); however, age-group analysis showed that this was only significant in the 30–39-year age group.
- In the intervention group, 19.8% of women diagnosed with cancer were found to have FIGO stage I, compared to 10.1% of women with cervical cancer in the control group ($p = 0.015$).
- In the intervention group there was a lower incidence of higher FIGO stage cancers (stage II or greater) among women 30–39 years of age, adjusted HR 0.51 (CI 0.29–0.92); no significant difference was seen overall among all age groups (Table 41.1).

Table 41.1 SUMMARY OF RESULTS

Outcome Rates (per 100,000 Person-Years)	Intervention	Control	Hazard Ratio Adjusted*
Cervical Cancer Incidence	60.9 ($n = 167$)	88.6 ($n = 158$)	0.75 (CI 0.59–0.95)
Incidence of ≥ Stage 2 Cancer	38.3 ($n = 105$)	54.9 ($n = 98$)	0.76 (CI 0.57–1.02)
Cervical Cancer Mortality	30.2 ($n = 83$)	51.5 ($n = 2$)	0.65 (CI 0.47–0.89)

* Adjusted for age, education, marital status, parity and cluster design

Criticisms and Limitations:

- Cause of death cannot always be determined accurately, as death records are often incomplete in rural India.
- Younger women <30 years of age were not included, and there was a heavy representation of women age 30–39, with women age 40–60 making up less than 50% of the total study population.
- It is difficult to establish and maintain quality assurance with VIA programs. This can make the sensitivity and specificity of VIA testing quite variable, with sensitivity ranging from 56% to 77% and specificity ranging from 64% to 86%.[2,3]

Other Relevant Studies and Information:

- Cytology-based cervical cancer screening programs have successfully reduced cervical cancer incidence in high-income countries, and now approximately 85% of cervical cancer deaths occur in low- and middle-income countries (LMICs), largely due to lack of screening and lack of human papillomavirus (HPV) vaccine access.[4] VIA using 3%–5% acetic acid is a low-cost way to screen for cervical dysplasia and treat during the same visit, reducing travel time, minimizing the number of visits, costs, and skilled labor requirements compared with cytology.
- Other studies have looked at visual inspection with Lugol's iodine (VILI) testing as an alternative screening method that has been shown to be more sensitive and specific for detecting Cervical Intraepithelial Neoplasia (CIN) 2 or higher,[5] but not as good as HPV testing. Additionally, Lugol's iodine is not as readily available as acetic acid (vinegar).
- Recent trials have shown that cervical HPV DNA testing is more sensitive for detecting CIN 2 and 3. In a randomized controlled trial comparing cervical DNA testing to vaginal DNA testing and VIA, cervical HPV testing was the most sensitive at 81.5%–85.3% (for CIN 2 and 3, respectively), followed by vaginal HPV testing at 69.6%–71.3%, and finally VIA ranging from 21.9% to 73.6%.[6] Rapid HPV testing is more objective and reproducible; however, costs may still be prohibitive in LMICs.[7]

Summary and Implications: In this analysis in resource-limited communities in India, screening, and if necessary treating, with VIA was shown to decrease both cervical cancer incidence and mortality. Though not as effective as standard cervical cancer screening with cervical cytology and HPV testing, VIA is an acceptable and cost-effective screening strategy for women age 30–59, at least until standard screening strategies such as HPV testing become more widely available in the developing world.

CLINICAL CASE: CERVICAL CANCER SCREENING IN LOW RESOURCE SETTINGS

Case Overview

The local government in a rural area of an LMIC is looking to improve cervical cancer incidence and mortality. There is no local pathology lab to interpret cytology due to prohibitive costs. They ask what the available options are for screening and prevention of cervical cancer, who the target audience should be, and how often to screen.

Suggested Answer

The above trial and discussion show that visual inspection with 3%–5% acetic acid (VIA) is an effective method for the detection and prevention of cervical cancer and decreases cervical cancer–related mortality in resource-denied countries. It can be performed by nonphysician clinicians after appropriate training. Patients who are VIA-positive undergo same-day cervical cryotherapy during which the abnormal cells are burned off. Efforts should be aimed at the younger age group of women (age 30–39), as this group was shown to have the highest benefit of cervical cancer incidence and mortality reduction thanks to VIA screening.

The World Health Organization (WHO) recommends that the general population undergo HPV DNA detection in a screen-and-treat approach starting at the age of 30 years, with regular screening every 5–10 years. Another option is the screen, triage, and treat approach, which consists of a primary screen using HPV DNA detection, which, if positive, is followed by triage tests such as VIA, colposcopy, cytology, or partial genotyping. Screening through this method should be performed every 5–10 years. Where HPV-based testing is not feasible and in settings where cytology is not available, WHO suggests a regular screening interval of every 3 years when using VIA as the primary screening test, among both the general population of women and women living with HIV.[3]

References

1. Sankaranarayanan R, Esmy PO, Rajkumar R, et al. Effect of visual screening on cervical cancer incidence and mortality in Tamil Nadu, India: A cluster-randomised trial. Lancet. 2007 Aug 4;370(9585):398–406. doi: 10.1016/S0140-6736(07)61195-7. PMID: 17679017.
2. Sankaranarayanan R, Basu P, Wesley RS, et al.; IARC Multicentre Study Group on Cervical Cancer Early Detection. Accuracy of visual screening for cervical neoplasia: Results from an IARC multicentre study in India and Africa. Int J Cancer. 2004 Jul 20;110(6):907–913. doi: 10.1002/ijc.20190. PMID: 15170675.
3. WHO Guideline for Screening and Treatment of Cervical Pre-Cancer Lesions for Cervical Cancer Prevention. 2nd ed. Geneva: World Health Organization; 2021.
4. de Martel C, Plummer M, Vignat J, Franceschi S. Worldwide burden of cancer attributable to HPV by site, country and HPV type. Int J Cancer. 2017 Aug 15;141(4): 664–670. doi: 10.1002/ijc.30716. PMID: 28369882; PMCID: PMC5520228.
5. Fokom-Domgue J, Combescure C, Fokom-Defo V, et al. Performance of alternative strategies for primary cervical cancer screening in sub-Saharan Africa: Systematic

review and meta-analysis of diagnostic test accuracy studies. *BMJ*. 2015 Jul 3;351:h3084. doi: 10.1136/bmj.h3084. PMID: 26142020; PMCID: PMC4490835.

6. Jeronimo J, Bansil P, Lim J, et al. A multicountry evaluation of careHPV testing, visual inspection with acetic acid, and papanicolaou testing for the detection of cervical cancer. *Int J Gynecol Cancer*. 2014;24(3):576–585. doi: 10.1097/IGC.0000000000000084

7. Pimple SA, Mishra GA. Optimizing high risk HPV-based primary screening for cervical cancer in low- and middle-income countries: Opportunities and challenges. *Minerva Ginecol*. 2019 Oct;71(5):365–371. doi: 10.23736/S0026-4784.19.04468-X. PMID: 31698891.

SECTION 6

Mental Health

In Section 6, Mental Health, we have included three studies highlighting the importance of primary care and community-based interventions in managing mental health in low-resource settings. These studies overlap with the Health Systems and Healthcare Delivery section, but they were separated to highlight the importance of mental health, which is often neglected and underfunded globally.

Can Community Health Workers Effectively Provide Cognitive Behavioral Therapy–Based Services?

REBECCA WHITE

In a poor rural community with little access to mental health care, integration of a cognitive behaviour therapy-based intervention into the routine work of community health workers more than halved the rate of depression in prenatally depressed women compared with those receiving enhanced routine care.[1]

Research Question: Can cognitive behavioral therapy delivered by community health workers to mothers with perinatal depression improve infant health outcomes?

Funding: Wellcome Trust

Year Study Began: 2005

Year Study Ended: 2007

Study Location: 40 sites in rural Pakistan

Who Was Included: Married women between the ages of 16–45 years in the third trimester of pregnancy, diagnosed with depression as determined by study psychiatrists.

Who Was Excluded: Women with a serious medical condition, a significant pregnancy-related illness, a substantial physical or learning disability, or a history of psychosis.

How Many Patients: 903

Study Overview: See Figure 42.1.

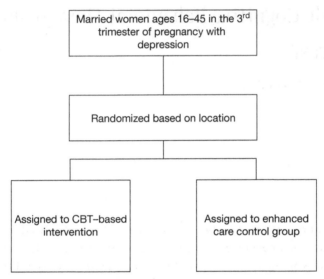

Figure 42.1. Overview of the study design.

Study Intervention: Study participants received visits from community health workers (CHWs) on an enhanced schedule with weekly visits in the last month of pregnancy, 3 visits in the first postpartum month, and then once a month visits for 9 months. Women in the intervention arm received cognitive behavioral therapy (CBT) based on the Thinking Health Program; those in the control arm received usual treatment at each visit.

Follow-Up: At 6 months and 1 year after delivery

Endpoints: Primary outcome: Infant height and weight at 6 months and 12 months.

Secondary outcomes: Depression and disability scores and contraceptive use at 12 months in mothers, and immunization rates and diarrhea 2 weeks prior to 1 year follow-up in infants.

RESULTS

- Depression and disability scores were nearly 50% lower in women in the intervention group compared with the control group at 12 months. These patients were also more likely to use contraception, and infants to mothers in the intervention group had improved health outcomes, including increased rate of completed immunizations and fewer diarrheal episodes 2 weeks prior to 12-month follow-up.
- Both mothers and fathers to infants in the intervention group reported significantly higher incidences of daily play with infants at 12 months.
- Nutritional indicators were not significantly different between intervention and control groups at 6 months or 12 months. In the intervention group, mothers whose depression had not remitted by 6 months had infants with significantly lower z-scores at 6 months and 12 months, compared with mothers who had recovered.
- Overall there were more underweight infants in both groups than the overall rate reported for Pakistan, likely because there was untreated maternal depression in both groups.

Table 42.1 OUTCOMES AT 12 MONTHS AFTER DELIVERY

Health Outcome	Intervention	Control	p Value
Depression score in mothers[*]	5.4	10.7	<0.0001
Disability score in mothers[†]	2.2	5.2	<0.0001
Height for age z-score in infants	−1.10	−1.36	0.07
Weight for age z-score in infants	−2.03	−2.16	0.37
Up-to-date infant immunizations	94%	85%	0.001
Maternal contraceptive use	62%	53%	0.002

[*] Mean Hamilton Depression Rating Scale; higher score indicates greater severity.
[†] Mean Brief Disability Questionnaire Score; higher score indicates greater disability.

Criticisms and Limitations: The intervention requires some level of mental health infrastructure that may not exist outside of trial settings, such as mental health supervisors, to provide ongoing training and support to non-specialist providers. The study authors suggest that peer supervision may be able to substitute for trained mental health workers for ongoing supervision and support; however, further studies would need to be conducted to determine efficacy of this level of supervision.

Other Relevant Studies and Information:

- Additional studies have shown that non-specialists have been able to effectively deliver evidence-based treatments in adults for depression, post-traumatic stress disorder (PTSD), and alcohol use disorders in low- and middle-income countries (LMICs).[2–4]
- Challenges in implementing mental health programs in LMICs include limited access to formally trained mental health professionals, emphasizing the need for informal and community-based mental health resources.[5]
- There is limited evidence available to support non-specialists delivering mental health interventions in children and adolescents[6] with a few studies showing mixed benefit for children with PTSD[7,8] and adolescents with depression.[9]

Summary and Implications: Some evidence-based mental health interventions that are typically delivered by trained mental health workers may be able to be effectively delivered by appropriately trained and supervised CHWs and other non-specialists. These interventions can be more readily implemented in settings where there is existing primary care infrastructure with community support.

CLINICAL CASE: COMMUNITY HEALTH WORKER BASED CBT FOR MANAGEMENT OF DEPRESSION IN RURAL AREAS

Case History

A 40-year-old female patient presents to a rural clinic with uncontrolled diabetes. She has had difficulty following her medication regimen and recommended diet. Upon further discussion, she also reports decreased mood and energy; she is sleeping more than she used to and does not feel motivated to work on improving her health. Depression screening suggests she has moderate depression. She has been receiving regular visits from her local community health worker for diabetes education and states that she enjoys those visits. There are no formal mental health services available in the immediate area and the patient is unable to travel to a larger city to receive counseling or depression treatment. In addition to addressing her uncontrolled diabetes, what community-based strategies could be implemented to improve her mental health and overall health outcomes?

Suggested Answer

Mental health treatment strategies often benefit from both collaborative care models (providers without formal mental health training consult those with formal training to provide this care to their patients) and community-based interventions, especially in areas with decreased access to formal mental health services. As this population already has a community health worker program that is integrated with the primary care clinic, implementing an evidence-based treatment program, such as a cognitive behavioral therapy–based intervention in patients with depression, may be an option. Obtain support for a potential program by discussing the observed problem with clinic leaders, the local CHWs, and influential community members for their observations, on-going challenges, community resources, and input on a strategy to address the problem. For successful implementation of CHW–based CBT service, consider what resources are required for initial training and ongoing supervision, including potential peer supervision among community health workers.

References

1. Rahman A, Malik A, Sikander S, Roberts C, Creed F. Cognitive behaviour therapy-based intervention by community health workers for mothers with depression and their infants in rural Pakistan: a cluster-randomised controlled trial. *Lancet*. 2008;372(9642):902–909. doi: 10.1016/S0140-6736(08)61400-2

2. Barnett ML, Gonzalez A, Miranda J, Chavira DA, Lau AS. Mobilizing community health workers to address mental health disparities for underserved populations: A systematic review. *Adm Policy Ment Health*. 2018;45(2):195–211. doi: 10.1007/s10488-017-0815-0

3. Sorsdahl K, Myers B, Ward CL, et al. Adapting a blended motivational interviewing and problem-solving intervention to address risky substance use amongst South Africans. *Psychother Res*. 2015;25(4):435–444. doi: 10.1080/10503307.2014.897770

4. Weiss WM, Murray LK, Zangana GAS, et al. Community-based mental health treatments for survivors of torture and militant attacks in Southern Iraq: A randomized control trial. *BMC Psychiatry*. 2015;15:249. doi: 10.1186/s12888-015-0622-7

5. Saraceno B, van Ommeren M, Batniji R, et al. Barriers to improvement of mental health services in low-income and middle-income countries. *Lancet*. 2007;370(9593):1164–1174. doi: 10.1016/S0140-6736(07)61263-X

6. van Ginneken N, Tharyan P, Lewin S, et al. Non-specialist health worker interventions for the care of mental, neurological and substance-abuse disorders in low- and middle-income countries. *Cochrane Database Syst Rev*. 2013;(11):CD009149. Published 2013 Nov 19. doi: 10.1002/14651858.CD009149.pub2

7. Tol WA, Komproe IH, Susanty D, Jordans MJD, Macy RD, De Jong JTVM. School-based mental health intervention for children affected by political violence in Indonesia: A cluster randomized trial. *JAMA*. 2008;300(6):655. doi: 10.1001/jama.300.6.655

8. Dawson K, Joscelyne A, Meijer C, Steel Z, Silove D, Bryant RA. A controlled trial of trauma-focused therapy versus problem-solving in Islamic children affected by civil conflict and disaster in Aceh, Indonesia. *Aust N Z J Psychiatry*. 2018;52(3):253–261. doi: 10.1177/0004867417714333

9. Bolton P, Bass J, Betancourt T, et al. Interventions for depression symptoms among adolescent survivors of war and displacement in northern Uganda: A randomized controlled trial. *JAMA*. 2007;298(5):519. doi: 10.1001/jama.298.5.519

43

Improving Mental Health Access Where There Is No Psychiatrist

Collaborative Care Model for Depression in Rural Nepal

RITI CHANDRASHEKHAR AND ANDREA WALKER

Our findings suggest that an adapted [collaborative care model] enhanced providers' perception and delivery of mental healthcare in our setting, and we observed improved clinical outcomes in patients with moderate or severe depression.[1]

—RIMAL ET AL.[1]

Research Question: Can collaborative care models (CoCMs) be effectively adapted in resource-constrained settings to expand access to high-quality mental healthcare?

Funding: National Institute of Mental Health, Harvard Medical School Center for Global Health Delivery, Dubai

Year Study Began: 2016

Year Study Published: 2021

Study Location: Achham, Nepal

Who Was Studied: Patients in the hospital's catchment area 15 years of age or older who were assessed at least once with a Patient Health Questionnaire-9

(PHQ-9) during the study period and scored moderate to severe unipolar depression at baseline (PHQ-9 score ≥10).

Who Was Excluded: Patients diagnosed with bipolar depression and patients who had a baseline PHQ-9 score <10 (suggesting mild or no depression).

How Many Patients: 201 patients

Study Overview: Figure 43.1 provides an overview of the study design, which focused on both provider experience and feedback with resultant changes to the CoCM, as well as monitoring patient outcomes.

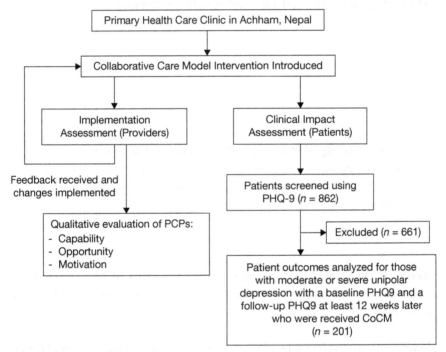

Figure 43.1. Overview of the study design.

Study Intervention: CoCM utilizes primary care providers (PCPs) and behavioral health providers such as social workers and counselors to evaluate and treat patients for mental health as a team. This shared treatment plan is developed and guided by a consultant psychiatrist. It should be noted that the psychiatrist does not perform direct patient care, but instead provides feedback to the non-specialist team. The CoCM model differs from a consultation or referral model since the psychiatrist specialist provides routine feedback on all mental health cases. Therefore the quality of supervision does not depend on the non-specialist's prioritization of specific patient cases.

Follow-Up: 12 weeks

Endpoints: Improvement in baseline PHQ9 scores of patients with moderate to severe unipolar depression scores.

RESULTS

- Qualitative data collected from the PCPs, behavioral health specialists, and consultant psychiatrist revealed the following:
  - All PCPs reported improved clinical knowledge and ability to identify and treat mental illness.
  - The team-based approach with counselors and the consultant psychiatrist improved their self-perceived competency. They also noted a positive change in their attitude about providing care for patients with mental illness, largely due to improved patient outcomes which improved their motivation.
- The comparison between post-intervention scores and baseline PHQ-9 scores was statistically significant (95% CI: 42%–56%). In essence, the scores obtained by patients post-intervention suggested a statistically significant decrease in their score.

Criticisms and Limitations: The primary limitation of this study is that there was not a control group, making it impossible to assess the true value of the program. In addition, this model is resource-intensive, potentially creating sustainability challenges.

Other Relevant Studies and Information:

- There is a disproportionate need for mental health care providers compared to those who are skilled to provide the service.[2] To address the shortage of mental health providers, CoCMs with indirect psychiatric patient evaluation through a PCP and behavioral health provider team have been promoted.
- The Improving Mood—Promoting Access to Collaborative Treatment (IMPACT) trial published in 2002 demonstrated a 50% greater improvement in depression treatment outcomes in the intervention group compared with the usual care group, with significant patient and primary care provider satisfaction.[3]

- Multiple studies show the effectiveness of CoCMs in improving mental health outcomes, although these studies were largely performed in high-income countries (HICs). One review of 79 RCTs of collaborative care for 24 308 participants of all ages with depression or anxiety demonstrated improvement in depression and anxiety outcomes.[4]

Summary and Implications: This study found that the CoCM is feasible to implement in LMICs and may be associated with improvement in outcomes for patients with depression. The findings also suggest the potential to adapt CoCMs to suit low resource settings within HICs.

CLINICAL CASE: USING THE COLLABORATIVE CARE MODEL TO INCREASE ACCESS TO MENTAL HEALTH CARE

Case History

You work in a hospital in a rural, low-resource district. There are no formally trained mental health providers, but there are some physicians and clinical officers working at a local hospital and clinic. Your district has recently implemented a community health worker program and you are required to improve access to mental health care services in a low resource setting. Based on this study and other proposed task-sharing models in this book, how could you address this problem?

Suggested Answer

The first suggested step would be to conduct a needs assessment. This will help identify the prevalence of mental health issues in the local population and thereby help prioritize the nature of mental health services required. Additionally, obtaining support for a potential program by discussing the observed problem with clinic leaders, the local community health workers, and influential community members will be vital.

The amalgamation of a primary care clinic resources and community health worker program might pave the way for scaling of CoCM that considers mental health services (refer the chapter "Can Community Health Workers Effectively Provide Cognitive Behavioral Therapy-Based Services"). For successful implementation of both programs, consider what resources are required for initial training and ongoing supervision, and be ready to accept feedback and be adaptable in your approach.

References

1. Rimal P, Choudhury N, Agrawal P, et al. Collaborative care model for depression in rural Nepal: A mixed-methods implementation research study. *BMJ Open*. 2021;11:e048481. doi: 10.1136/bmjopen-2020-048481.
2. Archer J, Bower P, Gilbody S, et al. Collaborative care for depression and anxiety problems. *Cochrane Database Syst Rev*. 2012;10:CD006525. Published 2012 Oct 17. doi: 10.1002/14651858.CD006525.pub2
3. Levine S, Unützer J, Yip JY, et al. Physicians' satisfaction with a collaborative disease management program for late-life depression in primary care. *Gen Hosp Psychiatry*. 2005; 27:383–391.
4. Unützer J, Katon W, Callahan CM, et al. Collaborative care management of late-life depression in the primary care setting: A randomized controlled trial. *JAMA*. 2002;288(22):2836–2845. doi: 10.1001/jama.288.22.2836

44

Nonphysician-Led Multidisciplinary Stepped-Care Program vs. Usual Primary Care Program for Females with Major Depression

SHAHEEN CHOWDHURY

We did not design the program to introduce radical changes to established practices. We aimed to improve existing care with structured protocols and rationalize the use of available resources.[1]

Research Question(s): Is a stepped-care program more effective than usual care in the primary-care management of depression in low-income women in Santiago, Chile?

Funding: US National Institute of Mental Health

Year Study Began: 2000

Year Study Published: 2003

Study Location: Santiago, Chile

Who Was Studied: Those who met the following criteria: female primary-care patients age 18–70 years with current DSM-IV major depressive illness; persistent depression as evidenced by a double-screening process 2 weeks apart.

Who Was Excluded: Patients with current psychotic symptoms, serious suicidal risk, history of mania, or current alcohol abuse; patients who had a psychiatric consultation or admission to hospital in the last 3 months.

How Many Patients: 240

Study Overview: See Figure 44.1.

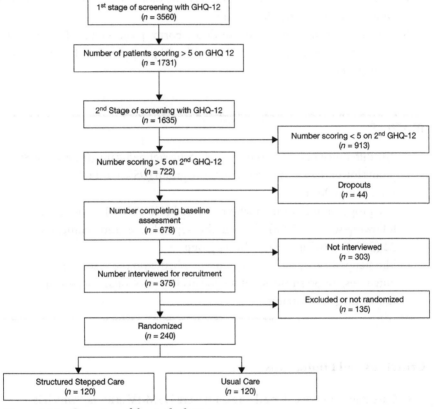

Figure 44.1. Overview of the study design.

Study Intervention: Study intervention was a multi-component, stepped-care program to improve treatment practices for depression and the efficiency in which resources are used. Stepped care consisted of a structured psychoeducational group, systematic monitoring of clinical progress, and a structured pharmaco-therapy program for patients with severe or persistent depression. It was led by trained nonphysician health workers. A doctor was involved only if medications were needed for patients with severe depression.

Participants in the usual care group received services from the primary care clinic, including referrals to the specialist and antidepressant treatment. Physicians treating the participants in the control group received guidelines on how to treat, and no services were withheld from the control group.

Follow-Up: 6 months.

Endpoints:

Primary outcome: Change in Hamilton Depression Rating Scores (HDRS) as continuous and categorical variables.

Secondary outcomes: 4 aspects of Short Form questionnaire (SF-36) sub-scales were used, which were mental health, emotional role, social functioning, and vitality.

RESULTS

- The difference in mean HDRS score of the stepped-care group was 8.89 points lower than that of the usual-care group (95% CI, 11.15–6.76 with *p*-value <0.0001).
- The proportion of women who recovered (HDRS <8) by 6-month follow-up was 73 (70%) of 104 in the stepped-care group compared with 32 (30%) of 107 in the usual-care group.
- The stepped-care group did significantly better on the secondary outcomes, SF-36 subscales of mental health, emotional role, social functioning, and vitality.

Criticisms and Limitations:

- Case definitions used for depression were DSM-IV criteria,[1] which is a specialist psychiatric construct that is difficult to translate to primary healthcare settings.[2]
- One of the most challenging aspects of treating depression in primary care is recognition of the disease, especially when the presenting complaints are nonspecific. In this study, the women studied were specifically screened for depression, which may be challenging to translate in real-world scenarios.

Other Relevant Studies and Information:

- The Lancet Commission on global mental health and sustainable development emphasized the importance of increased involvement of trained non-specialist mental health providers as well as patients in the provision of global mental health services.[3]
- A systematic review by Hoeft et al. on task-sharing in mental health concluded that task-sharing might facilitate reach and increase the effectiveness of mental healthcare in low-resource settings.[4]
- The MANAS study showed the effectiveness of nonphysician-led primary care–based interventions for common mental disorders including anxiety and depression.[5]
- Psychological interventions by non-specialist health workers were superior to enhanced usual care in treating depression and alcohol use disorder in primary care in India.[6]
- A meta-analysis of community-based psychosocial interventions for people with schizophrenia in low- and middle-income countries (LMICs) supports the effectiveness and feasibility of such interventions in schizophrenia.[7]
- A systematic review and meta-analysis found stepped care to be more effective in treatment of depressive disorders and at least as effective for anxiety disorders.[8]

Summary and Implications: This was a randomized controlled trial which compared the efficacy of a nonphysician-led structured stepped-care treatment program to usual primary care including referrals to specialists for the treatment of major depression in female patients. The significant improvement in the intervention group suggests that a stepped-care program empowering mid-level workers and increasing patient engagement can produce substantial gains in mental health, even in under-resourced settings.

CLINICAL CASE: MANAGEMENT OF DEPRESSION USING A NON-PHYSICIAN LED MULTI-DISCIPLINARY APPROACH

Case History
A 22-year-old female, Rupali, comes to your primary care clinic with complaints of a sensation of heaviness in her body and headaches for the last 3 months.

She has also been sleeping poorly and has a poor appetite. She attributes this to "weakness" secondary to complications that occurred after the birth of her second baby girl 5 months back. She denies any suicidal ideas, but says she sometimes wishes that she could fall asleep and not wake up until "her body felt better." She is accompanied by her aunt, who is a nurse at your facility and wonders if her niece is depressed. She also tells you that her niece is under a lot of stress at her in-laws' home where she lives.

You are worried about the possibility of depression and suicidal risk and you refer her to the psychiatrist in the nearby town.

On follow-up she reports that she was unable to communicate well with the psychiatrist as they did not speak the dialect that she is used to. She asks you if you had sent her to a "doctor for mental people" and reminds you that she has headache and body aches. She says that her family is no longer supportive of her treatment as they believe she is faking her symptoms. She says she was started on medication by the specialist but has not taken it as she did not believe it would help her.

You recently heard from her aunt that Rupali visited a local religious healer who is a leader in her community and now feels better with their interventions.

What systemic changes could have provided Rupali better care?

Suggested Answer

Locally based, systematic treatment is better than fragmented specialist care. More doctors and psychiatrists are often not the solution.

Rupali needed to be evaluated by someone who understood her context and psychosocial circumstances and their effect on her mental health. The religious community leader did, in fact, fill this role. They understood the pressure on Rupali to bear a son and were able to intervene on her behalf with her extended family, explaining the mind-body relationship in a culturally appropriate manner. They were also able to leverage social support for her when she disclosed to them that she was experiencing intimate partner violence. They suggested to her that she use antidepressant medication to address her sleep and appetite and give her body the best chance of recovery.

This is a role that needs to be systematized in local mental health programs.

References

1. Araya R, Rojas G, Fritsch R, et al. Treating depression in primary care in low-income women in Santiago, Chile: A randomised controlled trial. *Lancet*. 2003;361(9362): 995–1000.
2. Jacob KS, Patel V. Classification of mental disorders: A global mental health perspective. *Lancet*. 2014;383(9926):1433–1435.

3. Patel V, Saxena S, Lund C, et al. The Lancet Commission on global mental health and sustainable development. *Lancet*. 2018;392(10157):1553–1598.

4. Hoeft TJ, Fortney JC, Patel V, Unützer J. Task-sharing approaches to improve mental health care in rural and other low-resource settings: A systematic review. *J Rural Health*. 2018;34(1):48–62.

5. Patel V, Weiss HA, Chowdhary N, et al. Effectiveness of an intervention led by lay health counsellors for depressive and anxiety disorders in primary care in Goa, India (MANAS): A cluster randomised controlled trial. *Lancet*. 2010;376(9758):2086–2095.

6. Agabio R. Non-specialist health workers to treat excessive alcohol consumption and depression. *Lancet*. 2017;389(10065):133–135.

7. Asher L, Patel V, De Silva MJ. Community-based psychosocial interventions for people with schizophrenia in low and middle-income countries: systematic review and meta-analysis. *BMC Psychiatry*. 2017;17(1):355. Published 2017 Oct 30. doi: 10.1186/s12888-017-1516-7

8. Ho FY, Yeung WF, Ng TH, Chan CS. The Efficacy and Cost-Effectiveness of Stepped Care Prevention and Treatment for Depressive and/or Anxiety Disorders: A Systematic Review and Meta-Analysis. *Sci Rep*. 2016;6:29281. Published 2016 Jul 5. doi: 10.1038/srep29281

Noncommunicable Diseases

Although the burden of Noncommunicable Diseases (NCDs) is rising globally, Section 7 includes only three studies largely because NCD treatment is still an aspiration in many parts of the world. We have included one study on the use of aspirin in stroke as that is the most commonly available treatment, and one study on use Streptokinase in Acute myocardial infarction as cardiac catheterization is inaccessible in most parts of the world. Lastly, we have also included the SPRINT trial. As the management of hypertension is not generally resource-intensive, this chapter is meant to emphasize the importance of context in healthcare provision and how to responsibly adapt research from resource-abundant settings to resource-constrained settings.

Noncommunicable Diseases

45

Aspirin in Acute Stroke

When Thrombolysis Is Not Available

JESSICA BENDER

Study's Nickname: CAST (Chinese Acute Stroke Trial)
"Immediate treatment of acute ischaemic stroke with medium-dose aspirin (160 or 300mg daily) produces a modest, but definite ($2p = 0.001$), net reduction in early death or non-fatal stroke."[1]

Research Question: Does aspirin in the setting of acute ischemic stroke prevent short-term death and disability?

Funding: Medical Research Council helped fund the Clinical Trial Service Unit and Shandong Xinhua Pharmaceuticals donated trial tablets

Year Study Began: 1993

Year of Publication: 1997

Study Location: 413 Chinese hospitals

Who Was Studied: Patients with symptoms of presumed acute ischemic stroke, presenting within 48 hours to one of the participating hospitals. For comatose patients, a computed tomography (CT) scan was mandatory prior to participation.

Who Was Excluded: Patients with any contraindication to aspirin, as identified by the responsible physician. Contraindications included a history of bleeding gastric ulcer, allergy, low likelihood of benefit of hospitalization due to minor stroke, major life-threatening disease, or severe preexisting disability. Patients with a clear indication for aspirin, such as acute myocardial infarction, were also excluded.

How Many Patients: 21,106

Study Overview: See Figure 45.1

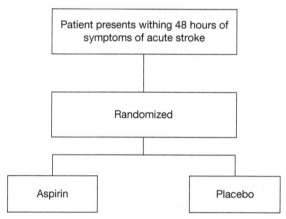

Figure 45.1. Summary of trial's design.

Study intervention: In this randomized controlled trial, participants in the intervention group received 160 mg of aspirin per day until hospital discharge, which was up to 4 weeks. Participants in the placebo group received a matching placebo tablet. The tablets were given by nasogastric feeding tube if the patient could not swallow. Other antiplatelet drugs or non-trial aspirin were not allowed unless a strong indication occurred after study enrollment, such as acute myocardial infarction.

Follow-Up: Until time of discharge, up to four weeks.

Endpoints: The primary endpoints were (1) death from any cause during 4 weeks and (2) death or dependence at time of discharge. Secondary endpoints included recurrent stroke, death, or non-fatal stroke during the treatment period, and additional major clinical events such as pulmonary embolism and hemorrhage.

RESULTS

- A 14% relative reduction in mortality was seen in the aspirin group (Table 45.1, 3.3% versus 3.9%) with a corresponding reduction in deaths of 5.4 per 1000 patients.

- At discharge, 30.5% of those receiving aspirin were dead or dependent compared to 31.6% receiving placebo, with a corresponding reduction in death or dependency of 13 per 1000 patients.
- There were fewer recurrent strokes in the aspirin group compared to placebo (3.2% versus 3.4%) although this difference was not statistically significant ($p > 0.1$).
- There were fewer recurrent ischemic strokes in the aspirin group (1.6% vs. 2.1%) but more hemorrhagic strokes (1.1% vs. 0.9%).
- The combined endpoint of death or non-fatal stroke at 4 weeks was 5.3% in the aspirin group compared to 5.9% in the placebo group.

Table 45.1 SUMMARY OF CAST's MAIN FINDINGS

Outcome	Aspirin Group	Placebo Group	*P* value
Death during treatment period	3.3%	3.9%	0.04
Death or dependency at time of discharge	30.5%	31.6%	0.08
Recurrent ischemic stroke	1.6%	2.1%	0.01
Recurrent hemorrhagic stroke	1.1%	0.9%	>0.1
Death or non-fatal stroke at 4 weeks	5.3%	5.9%	0.03

Criticisms and Limitations:

- Responsible physicians excluded patients based on their perception of low likelihood of benefit of aspirin, which may have included the presence of a very minor stroke, a massive stroke, other life-threatening disease, or preexisting disability. These exclusions may contribute to sampling bias and could limit the applicability of the results.
- Only 12% of participants did not undergo CT scan prior to randomization, which may limit applicability of the results to patients in hospitals without access to CT scan.
- In some areas of the world, presentation to care may be delayed beyond the 48 hours used in CAST.

Other Relevant Studies:

- The International Stroke Trial (IST) was a randomized, open trial of antithrombotic therapy including aspirin within 48 hours of acute ischemic stroke.[2] IST was conducted in 36 countries at the same time as CAST and also showed aspirin led to a reduction in death or recurrent stroke at 14 days. At 6 months, IST showed that acute use of aspirin led to a statistically nonsignificant trend toward decreased death or dependency.

- Subgroup analysis of IST and CAST showed those without CT imaging prior to aspirin still had better outcomes than those in the placebo arm, suggesting that the benefit of aspirin use acutely may outweigh the risk of intracranial hemorrhage, even without imaging to rule out haemorrhagic stroke.[3]
- As of the 2013 Global Burden of Disease study, stroke was the second largest contributor to age-adjusted disability-adjusted life years (DALYs) in developing countries.[4] Hemorrhagic stroke was a larger contributor to DALYs and mortality compared to ischemic stroke in developing countries.
- The most recent American Heart Association/American Stroke Association guidelines recommend aspirin initiation within 24–48 hours of ischemic stroke based on the results of CAST and IST.[5]

Summary and Implications: CAST was one of the first large studies to show a benefit of aspirin in the acute post-stroke period. Aspirin results in a modest reduction in disability and death when given in the acute period after presumed ischemic stroke.

The high burden of stroke and subsequent loss of DALYs in the Global South suggests that aspirin use in acute stroke is a worthwhile intervention. Aspirin should not be used acutely if hemorrhagic stroke is suspected, and differentiating hemorrhagic versus ischemic stroke may be challenging without access to computed tomography scan.

CLINICAL CASE: MANAGEMENT OF ACUTE STROKE IN LOW RESOURCE SETTINGS WHERE ADVANCED DIAGNOSTICS AND THERAPEUTICS ARE NOT AVAILABLE

Case History

A 45-year-old woman presents to a clinic in southeastern Liberia with weakness. While working on a farm 4 days prior, she developed sudden onset slurred speech and right arm weakness. After a day of persistent symptoms, her family started to collect money for transportation to the clinic, but flooded roads prevented her from leaving the village for another 2 days. On presentation to the clinic, she reports no headache, neck stiffness, seizure, or vomiting.

Her blood pressure is 155/90. She is awake with expressive dysphasia and 3/5 strength in her right arm. Point of care glucose is 85 and malaria rapid diagnostic test is negative. No other diagnostics are available at the clinic. Based on the results of CAST, should she receive aspirin?

Suggested Answer

She should receive aspirin. Although she is already out of the 48-hour acute window that was used in CAST, there is likely still some benefit of aspirin in preventing near-term death and dependency. This case illustrates some of the potential delays in accessing care, particularly in rural areas. This case also illustrates the problem of lack of access to head imaging to definitively rule out hemorrhagic stroke before aspirin initiation. Certain clinical characteristics, such as this patient's lack of seizure, headache, neck stiffness, and coma, plus a diastolic blood pressure under 110 mmHg, may be useful in predicting ischemic versus hemorrhagic stroke.[6] Additional delays in receiving aspirin may occur due to delay in transportation from clinic to hospital or supply chain problems leading to stock-outs of aspirin in more rural areas.

References

1. CAST: Randomised placebo-controlled trial of early aspirin use in 20,000 patients with acute ischaemic stroke. CAST (Chinese Acute Stroke Trial) Collaborative Group. *Lancet.* 1997;349(9066):1641–1649.
2. The International Stroke Trial (IST): A randomised trial of aspirin, subcutaneous heparin, both, or neither among 19435 patients with acute ischaemic stroke. International Stroke Trial Collaborative Group. *Lancet.* 1997;349(9065):1569–1581.
3. Chen ZM, Sandercock P, Pan HC, et al. Indications for early aspirin use in acute ischemic stroke: A combined analysis of 40 000 randomized patients from the chinese acute stroke trial and the international stroke trial. On behalf of the CAST and IST collaborative groups. *Stroke.* 2000;31(6):1240–1249. doi: 10.1161/01.str.31.6.1240
4. Feigin VL, Krishnamurthi RV, Parmar P, et al. Update on the Global Burden of Ischemic and Hemorrhagic Stroke in 1990–2013: The GBD 2013 Study. *Neuroepidemiology.* 2015;45(3):161–176. doi: 10.1159/000441085
5. Powers WJ, Rabinstein AA, Ackerson T, et al. Guidelines for the early management of patients with acute ischemic stroke: 2019 Update to the 2018 guidelines for the early management of acute ischemic stroke: A guideline for healthcare professionals from the American Heart Association/American Stroke Association [published correction appears in Stroke. 2019 Dec;50(12):e440-e441]. *Stroke.* 2019;50(12):e344–e418. doi: 10.1161/STR.0000000000000211
6. Runchey S, McGee S. Does this patient have a hemorrhagic stroke?: Clinical findings distinguishing hemorrhagic stroke from ischemic stroke. *JAMA.* 2010;303(22):2280–2286. doi: 10.1001/jama.2010.754

46

Unavailability of Cardiac Catheterization

Thrombolysis Is Safe and Effective in Myocardial Infarction

PETER OLDS

> . . . streptokinase and aspirin are practicable, and are of demonstrated value and safety. If both are used widely then they should avoid several tens of thousands of deaths each year.
>
> —ISIS-2 INVESTIGATORS[1]

Research Question: To evaluate the effect of streptokinase and aspirin, alone and in combination, on vascular mortality in patients with acute myocardial infarction (MI).

Funding: Behringwerke, a subsidiary of Hoechst (manufacturers of Streptase [streptokinase]). Aspirin and its placebo were donated by Sterling Drugs.

Year Study Began: 1985

Year Study Published: 1988

Study Location: 417 hospitals in 16 countries (Australia, Austria, Belgium, Canada, Denmark, Finland, France, Germany, Ireland, New Zealand, Norway, Spain, Sweden, Switzerland, United Kingdom, United States)

Who Was Studied: Patients up to 24 hours after onset of suspected acute MI and where the physician was uncertain if streptokinase or aspirin were indicated.

Who Was Excluded: Those with contraindications to streptokinase or aspirin:
- *Absolute contraindications*: any history of stroke or gastrointestinal (GI) hemorrhage or ulcer.
- *Relative contraindications*: recent arterial puncture, recent severe trauma, severe persistent hypertension, allergy to streptokinase or aspirin, low risk of cardiac death, or some other life-threatening disease.

How Many Patients: 17 187

Study Overview: See Figure 46.1.

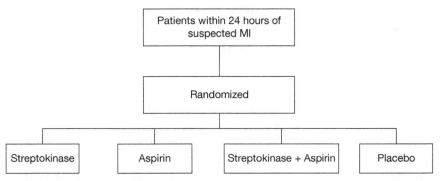

Figure 46.1. Overview of the study design.

Study Intervention: Patients were randomized by two-by-two factorial design to receive either a 1-hour IV infusion of 1.5 MU of streptokinase, 1 month of 160 mg/day enteric-coated aspirin, both treatments, or neither.

Follow-Up: Maximum total follow-up of 34 months with median of 15 months

Endpoints:
  Primary outcome: Vascular mortality at 5 weeks and entire follow-up period (median 15 months).
  Secondary outcomes: Nonfatal reinfarction, bleeds requiring transfusion, nonfatal strokes, cerebral hemorrhage.

RESULTS

- Streptokinase reduced the odds of 5-week mortality by 25% compared with those receiving placebo infusions (9.2 vs. 12%) (Table 46.1).
- Aspirin reduced the odds of 5-week mortality by 23% compared with those receiving placebo tablets (9.4 vs. 11.8%).

- The combination of aspirin and streptokinase led to a 42% reduction in the odds of mortality at 5 weeks compared with those receiving both placebos (8.0 vs. 13.2%).
- The effects of aspirin and streptokinase were largely independent of each other: streptokinase reduced mortality in both aspirin and placebo groups (28% and 23% reductions, respectively), and aspirin reduced mortality in both streptokinase and placebo groups (25% and 21% reductions, respectively).
- When compared with placebo, the combination of aspirin and streptokinase led to:
  - Slight increases in major bleeding (0.6% vs. 0.3%, $2P < 0.001$) and hemorrhagic strokes (0.1% and 0.0%, $2P < 0.02$)
  - A halving of nonfatal strokes (0.3% vs. 0.6%, $2P = 0.02$)
- Aspirin reduced the reinfarction rate by 50% (1.0% vs. 2.0%)

Table 46.1 SUMMARY OF ISIS-2 RESULTS

Intervention	5-Week Mortality vs. Placebo (%)	Relative Risk (RR)	Number Needed to Treat (NNT)	2P Value
Streptokinase	9.2 vs. 12.0	0.77	35	<0.00001
Aspirin	9.4 vs. 11.8	0.80	42	<0.00001
Streptokinase + Aspirin	8.0 vs. 13.2	0.60	19	<0.0001

Criticisms and Limitations:

- The study is criticized for the fact that it lacked proper equipoise regarding thrombolytic therapy in acute MI. Despite a large meta-analysis showing significant mortality benefit with thrombolytics in acute MI, expert opinion at the time was divided and the study was allowed to proceed.
- The primary limitation of ISIS-2 is that the study population is not globally representative. Women are underrepresented, making up only 23% of study participants, and all study sites are in the Global North and thus the study population is likely overrepresented with white/ Caucasian participants (this is inferred, since ISIS-2 does not provide a breakdown of participants by race).

Other Relevant Studies and Information:

- Follow-up meta-analysis of over 200,000 patients showed that aspirin's benefits extend to non-ST-elevation myocardial infarction (NSTEMI) and unstable angina (UA), reducing rates of nonfatal MI, nonfatal stroke, or vascular death by 46% in UA and 30% in MI.[2]

- Further studies have shown that dual antiplatelet therapy, with aspirin and a P2Y12 inhibitor (clopidogrel), was safe and significantly lowered mortality in patients with acute coronary syndrome (ACS).[3]
- Although there are no high-quality randomized controlled trials testing the efficacy of thrombolysis in MI in the Global South, it is the most common mode of treatment available in low- and middle-income countries (LMICs).[4]
- Importantly, acute hospital care is only one part of acute MI care. Pre-hospital identification, triaging, and treatment, as well as post-hospital longitudinal care, are critical to improving survival.
- Mortality for acute MI remains unacceptably high in low-resource settings, highlighting the dire need for better pre-hospital care, effective hospital management, and improved access to percutaneous coronary intervention (PCI).[5]

Summary and Implications: In patients who present with acute MI, strepto-kinase infusion combined with 1 month of aspirin reduces vascular mortality by 40%, including reductions in overall strokes and re-infarction. This combination was generally safe, with small increases in major bleeding and cerebral hemorrhage. Thrombolytic treatment remains a preferred approach for managing ACS in resource limited settings where cardiac catheterization is not readily available.

CLINICAL CASE: MANAGEMENT OF ST ELEVATION MYOCARDIAL INFARCTION WITH STREPTOKINASE

Case History
A 54-year-old woman presents with substernal chest pain with radiation to her epigastrium. She has a history of gastritis. Vitals show a temperature of 36.9C, HR of 103 bpm, BP 160/88 mmHg, RR 18 rpm, and SpO2 98% on room air. ECG is consistent with an anterior ST-segment elevation MI.

1. What information do you need from this patient to assess the benefit of streptokinase?
2. When would you not give streptokinase?

3. Your facility doesn't have streptokinase. What benefit would aspirin alone provide to this patient?
4. Is there a benefit to further antiplatelet therapy?
5. Your site does not have an ECG. How do you proceed?

Suggested Answers

1. Time since symptoms onset (if less than 24 hours ago).
2. If symptom onset was >24 hours prior, or if the patient has any absolute contraindications to streptokinase (severe hypertension, recent stroke, etc.).
3. Aspirin would reduce the odds of mortality by 23% and halves the risk of reinfarction or stroke.
4. Dual antiplatelet therapy (DAPT) with aspirin and P2Y12 inhibitor (i.e., clopidogrel) is safe and reduces mortality, reinfarction, and stroke.
5. This is sadly a very common scenario in low-resource settings. Given its efficacy and safety, a loading dose of aspirin (160–325 mg) is first-line therapy in patients with presumed ACS. Due to the rising prevalence of heart disease around the world, your medical facility should be prepared for patients who have a high suspicion for ACS. In synthesizing your facility's resources, population disease prevalence, and clinical suspicion, your team should develop a framework for how to approach cases of presumed ACS, considering when to add PY12 inhibitor and when to transfer patients to higher levels of care.

References

1. ISIS-2 Collaborative Group. Randomised trial of intravenous streptokinase, oral aspirin, both, or neither among 17187 cases of suspected acute myocardial infarction. *Lancet.* 1988;332(8607):349–360.
2. Antithrombotic Trialists' Collaboration. Collaborative meta-analysis of randomised trials of antiplatelet therapy for prevention of death, myocardial infarction, and stroke in high risk patients [published correction appears in BMJ 2002 Jan 19;324(7330):141]. *BMJ.* 2002;324(7329):71–86. doi:10.1136/bmj.324.7329.71
3. Mehta SR, Yusuf S, Peters RJ, et al. Effects of pretreatment with clopidogrel and aspirin followed by long-term therapy in patients undergoing percutaneous coronary intervention: the PCI-CURE study. *Lancet.* 2001;358(9281):527–533. doi: 10.1016/s0140-6736(01)05701-4

4. Yao H, Ekou A, Niamkey T, et al. Acute coronary syndromes in sub-Saharan Africa: A 10-year systematic review. *J Am Heart Assoc.* 2022 Jan 4;11(1):e021107. doi: 10.1161/JAHA.120.021107. PMID: 34970913.

5. Fanta K, Daba FB, Asefa ET, et al. Management and 30-Day Mortality of Acute Coronary Syndrome in a Resource-Limited Setting: Insight From Ethiopia. A Prospective Cohort Study. *Front Cardiovasc Med.* 2021;8:707700. Published 2021 Sep 17. doi: 10.3389/fcvm.2021.707700

47

SPRINT Trial

Hypertension Management in Resource-Denied Settings

TIMOTHY S. LAUX

... targeting a systolic blood pressure of less than 120 mmHg, as compared with less than 140 mmHg, resulted in lower rates of fatal and nonfatal major cardiovascular events and death ... although significantly higher rates of some adverse events were observed....

—SPRINT RESEARCH GROUP[1]

Research Question(s): Is there any difference in cardiovascular outcomes between intensive systolic blood pressure (SBP) goal (SBP <120 mmHg) or a more lenient goal (SBP <140 mmHg) in hypertensive patients without diabetes?

Funding: Multiple US government agencies

Year Study Began: 2010

Year Study Published: 2015

Study Location: 102 clinical sites in the United States

Who Was Studied: Those who met all of the following criteria:
- ≥50 years old
- Baseline SBP criteria based on the number of medications each individual was already taking

- Increased cardiovascular risk (≥1 one of the following):
  - Cardiovascular disease (except previous stroke)
  - Chronic kidney disease (CKD) with an eGFR of 20 to 60 mL/min/ 1.73 m^2 of body surface area (BSA)
  - >15% cardiovascular disease risk (per Framingham score)
  - ≥75 years old.

Who Was Excluded:
- <50 years old
- Previous stroke or dementia
- Diabetes mellitus
- Malignant hypertension
- Polycystic kidney disease
- Assisted-living facility residents or life expectancy <3 years.

How Many Patients: 9361

Study Overview: See Figure 47.1.[1]

Eligibility	Randomization	Loss to Follow-Up	Analyzed
14 692 assessed	9361 (63.8%) randomized, 4678 to intensive arm, 4683 to standard arm	986 lost to follow-up (10.5%), 489 from intensive arm, 497 from standard arm	9361 analyzed (intention-to-treat)

Figure 47.1. Overview of the study design.

Study Intervention: Patients were randomized to the intensive (SBP goal <120 mmHg) or standard group (SBP <140 mmHg). Per previous trials, protocols encouraged starting with a 2- (or 3-) drug regimen, including a thiazide diuretic and/or an ACE inhibitor (ACEi)/angiotensin receptor blocker (ARB) and/or a calcium channel blocker (CCB).

Follow-Up: Stopped early at a median follow-up of 3.26 years.

Endpoints: Primary outcome: composite outcome of myocardial infarction, other acute coronary syndromes, stroke, heart failure, or death (from a cardio-vascular cause). Study also included multiple secondary outcomes, notably all-cause mortality, worsening renal disease, and serious adverse events from study medications.

RESULTS

- The study intervention allowed for rapid and sustained differences in SBP between the two intervention groups (121.5 mmHg in the intensive group, 134.6 mmHg in the standard group).
- The trial was terminated early due to prespecified safety analyses. At that time, the number needed to treat (NNT) for the primary composite outcome was 61, while the NNT for all-cause mortality was 90. These approximated the number needed to harm (NNH) for eGFR reduction in patients without baseline CKD (38), hypotension (107), or syncope (173).
- A difference in rates of the primary outcome occurred after ~12 months, while a difference in all-cause mortality became apparent after ~24 months.
- Serious adverse events were common in both groups (intensive: 1793 participants [38.3%]; standard: 1736 participants [37.1%]). When serious adverse events were analyzed for a likely link to the intervention, the difference was statistically significant.

Criticisms and Limitations:

- The prolonged time until a difference in various outcomes leads to concerns about external validity in many settings where 12 to 24 months of follow-up and adherence are difficult.
- Even in lower-resourced settings where 12 to 24 months of consistent follow-up are possible, the intervention arm required (on average) 2.8 medications per participant. This may not only prove onerous for over-stretched supply chains, but also lead to poor medication adherence.
- SPRINT inclusion criteria were fairly restrictive. Notably, the trial excluded the frail elderly, a population in whom there is substantial debate about blood pressure goals.

Other Relevant Studies and Information:

- ACCORD[2]—Blood pressure goal in type 2 diabetics. Rates of major cardiovascular events were similar between intensive (SBP <120 mmHg) or standard (SBP <140 mmHg) arms. Rates of stroke (a secondary analysis) were lower in the intensive arm.
- SPS3 Trial[3]—Blood pressure goals in patients with prior stroke. Rates of recurrent strokes were similar between intensive (SBP <130 mmHg)

and standard (SBP <150 mmHg) arms. There were lower rates of hemorrhagic stroke in the intensive arm.

- A large meta-analysis[4] (involving ~45 000 patients) showed a similar overall pattern of results with intensive blood pressure control (decreased major cardiovascular events and strokes but more severe hypotension), despite much smaller absolute differences in SBP (6.8 mmHg) and DBP (3.5 mmHg).
- Participants enrolled in the SPRINT Trial were followed for patient-reported outcomes. There were no significant differences.[5]

Summary and Implications: In the setting of a randomized controlled trial, intensive blood pressure control more effectively meets clinical endpoints but only after 1–2 years of treatment and with high rates of worrisome adverse events (that start happening immediately). How well this translates to real-world settings—especially in lower-resourced settings—is up for debate and likely requires a deep knowledge of local contexts for appropriate application.

CLINICAL CASE: CONTROL OF HYPERTENSION IN RESOURCE DENIED SETTINGS IN THE CONTEXT OF SPRINT TRIAL

Case History

A 58-year-old male with a history of hypertension complicated by chronic kidney disease (CKD) stage IIIb is referred to your care by a community health worker (CHW) from a remote, rural community.

This gentleman is well known to his CHW as someone intermittently on medications due to his work as a migrant laborer. When last seen, he had returned from working and his BP (off medicines) was 175/100 mmHg. Today, his blood pressure is 160/90. His A1c is 5.3%.

He reports that he does try to take his medicines when working but runs out when away for longer than expected.

He reports his father had high blood pressure and passed abruptly. He is aware that his blood pressure is elevated and would like to lower it.

Suggested Answer

This is a good setting for a discussion about risks and benefits and shared decision-making. After all, the benefits seen in the SPRINT Trial take 1 year to accrue, but the adverse events can occur immediately. A good place to start might be problem-solving how best to make sure he does not run out of medications while working. Once addressed, given his remote home and inability to monitor for adverse events related to intensive control (notably electrolyte and renal issues), consider starting any medication that is effective and dosed daily with a goal SBP of <140 mmHg.

If, over time and in the setting of a growing therapeutic relationship, it becomes clear that the patient is not experiencing any side effects and is finding ways to adhere to his medicines, he may be a candidate for a more intensive SBP goal of <120 mmHg. However, initially, the risks likely outweigh the benefits and other eventualities must be addressed prior to more intensive care.

References

1. Wright JT, Jr., Williamson JD, Whelton PK, et al. A randomized trial of intensive versus standard blood-pressure control. *N Engl J Med.* 2015;373:2103–2116.
2. Cushman WC, Evans GW, Byington RP, et al. Effects of intensive blood-pressure control in type 2 diabetes mellitus. *N Engl J Med.* 2010;362:1575–1585.
3. Benavente OR, Coffey CS, Conwit R, et al. Blood-pressure targets in patients with recent lacunar stroke: The SPS3 randomised trial. *Lancet.* 2013;382:507–515.
4. Xie X, Atkins E, Lv J, et al. Effects of intensive blood pressure lowering on cardiovascular and renal outcomes: Updated systematic review and meta-analysis. *Lancet.* 2016;387:435–443.
5. Berlowitz DR, Foy CG, Kazis LE, et al. Effect of intensive blood-pressure treatment on patient-reported outcomes. *N Engl J Med.* 2017;377:733–744.

SECTION 8

Surgery

Section 8, Global Surgery, incorporates three studies that focus on lifesaving measures in the field. Ketamine is a commonly used deep-sedation anesthetic that is useful when general anesthesia is not available to perform lifesaving procedures. Task shifting for C-sections, one of the most critical lifesaving surgeries, is a common approach to improving patient access to care. Surgical checklists are low-cost interventions recommended by the WHO and are proven to reduce surgical morbidity and mortality.

48

Where There Is No Anesthetist, Is Ketamine a Good Alternative?

NAMAN SHAH

The Every Second Matters (ESM)-Ketamine package was safe and feasible and expanded access to emergency and essential surgery in rural Kenya when no anesthetist was available[1]

—BURKE ET AL.[1]

Research Question: Can a ketamine-based protocol for emergency and essential procedures that is implemented by non-anesthetists provide safe and effective anesthesia?

Funding: Multiple donor agencies, including: Ujenzi Charitable Trust; Elrha's Research for Health in Humanitarian Crises (R2HC) Program and the Saving Lives at Birth Partners; United States Agency for International Development; Government of Norway; Bill & Melinda Gates Foundation; Grand Challenges Canada; UK Government; and Korea International Cooperation Agency. The R2HC program is funded equally by the Wellcome Trust and the Department for International Development (DfID).

Year Study Began: 2013

Year Study Published: 2017

Study Location: 15 facilities across Siaya, Homa Bay, Garissa, and Mandera counties, Kenya

Who Was Studied: Patients who presented to an "active" project hospital when either an anesthetist was unavailable and patient transfer was not possible or would result in harm; the procedure would have not been previously performed by an anesthetist; or the patient could not afford the anesthetist charges.

Who Was Excluded: None

How Many Patients: 1216

Study Overview: See Figure 48.1.

Study Intervention: Each study site selected 2 or more staff (nurses, clinical officers, or physicians) to undergo a 5-day ESM-Ketamine training. Sites were supplied with kits of necessary supplies, along with wall charts and pocket charts modeled after the Safe Surgery checklist. Patients enrolled into the study received a preoperative assessment, including completion of the ESM-Ketamine checklist by a trained provider. Routine anesthesia measures including vital signs, intravenous catheterization, pre-oxygenation, and use of pulse oximetry and blood pressure monitoring devices were applied. Anesthesia was then induced with intravenous ketamine at a dose 1–2 mg/kg with additional doses of 0.25 mg–2 mg/kg every 10–15 minutes as needed for the maintenance of anesthesia. Adjunct medicines included the use of diazepam, promethazine, or prochlorperazine, and atropine for hallucinations and agitation, nausea, and hypersalivation, respectively, as needed. Recovery to pretreatment levels of verbalization, awareness, and muscular activity was monitored by the ESM-Ketamine provider. There was no control group in this study.

Follow-Up: 2 weeks

Endpoints:
  Primary outcome: Safety represented by all adverse events (AE). Hallucinations and/or agitation treated with diazepam and brief periods (SpO2 <92% for <30 s) of intraoperative hypoxia were classified as AEs. Ketamine-related deaths or injuries and prolonged periods (>30 s) of intraoperative hypoxia were classified as serious AEs.
  Secondary outcomes: Feasibility consisting of demand, acceptability, and practicality of the ESM-Ketamine package, assessed through key-informant semi-structured interviews.

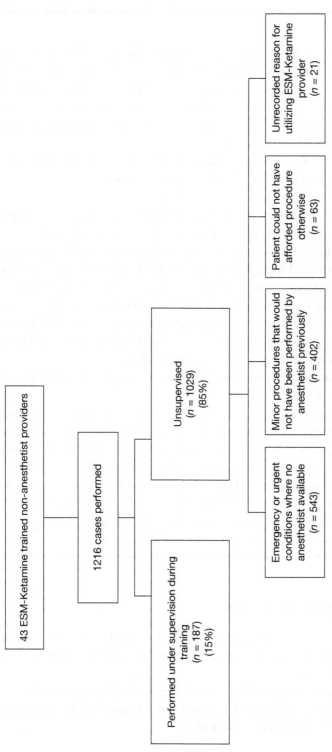

Figure 48.1. Summary of the ESM-Ketamine study population.

RESULTS

- Among ESM-Ketamine supported procedures, 518 (43%) were obstetric or gynecologic, 429 (35%) general surgery, 192 (16%) orthopedic, and 77 (6%) head and neck cases. Of these, 269 cases (22%) met the Lancet Commission definition of Bellwether Procedures such as emergency cesarean sections, emergency laparotomies, and open fracture repairs.
- Adverse events (AEs) included:
  - 3.2% of patients experienced brief hypoxia (<30 seconds), and 13% of patients experienced hallucination or agitation.
- Severe adverse events (SAEs) included:
  - 0.6% of patients experienced prolonged hypoxia, and 0.3% of patients died due to any cause, but none was attributed to ketamine.
  - Among the prolonged oxygen desaturation cases, 4 were associated with ESM-Ketamine training violations, including rapid administration of ketamine, failure to pre-oxygenate, and excessive diazepam dose. After a refresher training, there were no further such events. Two cases were due to airway obstructions which were recovered with basic anesthesia skills, and one case was due to the absence of peripheral pulses due to severe maternal hemorrhage.
- The incidence of AEs and SAEs was not correlated with the ketamine dose that was used.
- Key informants ($n = 27$) included ESM-Ketamine providers, surgeons, and hospital administrators and provided four main themes: (1) the wide availability and low cost of ketamine helped with the financial burden of surgeries; (2) the intervention decreased waiting times, increased surgical capacity, and improved the reputation of facilities and perception of quality of care; (3) ESM-Ketamine improved job satisfaction for trained providers; and (4) the intervention was best in surgical emergencies as a second-line option only if no anesthetist was available.

Criticisms and Limitations:

- This study may not be generalizable. The specific context, including the age and types of cases and prior skills of providers, may or may not apply elsewhere.
- There was no control group in this study, which either would not have been ethical and perhaps even legal through randomization, or comparable through observation.

- This study raises considerations about the trade-offs between putting resources into the development of formal anesthesia services versus putting resources into task-shifting.[2–4]

Other Relevant Studies and Information: The safe use of ketamine by non-anesthetists is supported by several other studies by this group and others.[2,5,6] Some key supporting information includes fetal outcomes during use in obstetric surgery, where no concerns were found,[7] as well as patient surveys of intraoperative awareness and experience, which were overwhelmingly favorable.[8]

Ketamine was approved by the FDA as an anesthetic in 1970 and has been on the World Health Organization's Essential Medicines List since 1985. In spite of recent concerns in some countries about its potential as a drug of abuse, the WHO has reiterated that ketamine should not be controlled under international conventions due to its essential role in surgery in low-resource countries.

Summary and Implications: The ESM-Ketamine package implemented across a range of hospitals and providers in rural Kenya was safe and feasible. The intervention expanded access to emergency and essential surgery. Expanding ketamine-based anesthetic training and programs could help ensure safe anesthesia services when an anesthetist is not available. Ketamine use may not be appropriate for complex or prolonged surgeries or intra-abdominal surgery, where muscle relaxation is necessary, without the use of additional techniques.

CLINICAL CASE: KETAMINE ANESTHESIA FOR ESSENTIAL SURGERY BY NON-ANESTHETISTS

Case History
A 24-year-old G4P3 mother in rural India has been laboring at home for more than 2 days before presenting to the hospital for obstruction of labor. On exam the patient has a heart rate of 122, blood pressure of 120/84, term abdomen, present fetal heart tones, and a fully dilated cervix, head at −2 station with thick caput. Emergency surgery is indicated for delivery and a trained provider is available. However, the sole anesthetist at the hospital is out of town and the nearest referral center is at least 3 hours away. Based on the results of the ESM-Ketamine study, would the use of ketamine be an appropriate alternative?

Suggested Answer
The ESM-Ketamine study showed that with minimal training, a range of clinical providers could safely and effectively provide anesthetic services where no

anesthetist was available. Ketamine is often ideal for the surgery of shock and sepsis, as it does not decrease cardiac output or vascular tone. Additionally, ketamine maintains the respiratory drive and does not require the use of an advanced airway. Common side effects of ketamine included hallucinations, agitation, or hypersalivation, and were easily managed. Serious adverse events were rare and were effectively managed using basic anesthesia skills.

The patient in this vignette is typical of patients included in the ESM-Ketamine study. Emergency cesarean section represents a common indication in this case series and is the most commonly conducted essential surgery globally. In the absence of ketamine, the delay in care could have disastrous consequences for both fetal and maternal well-being, as well as the possibility of financial impoverishment of the family. The inability to manage the patient would also affect the physician's morale and the reputation of the hospital within the community. Thus, she should undergo the indicated operation in a timely and safe manner provided that a ketamine-trained provider and the basic supporting anesthesia resources are available.

References

1. Burke TF, Suarez S, Senay A, et al. Safety and feasibility of a ketamine package to support emergency and essential surgery in Kenya when no anesthetist is available: An analysis of 1216 consecutive operative procedures. *World J Surg.* 2017 Dec;41(12):2990–2997. doi: 10.1007/s00268-017-4312-0

2. Burke TF, Suarez S, Senay A, et al. Safety and feasibility of a ketamine package to support emergency and essential surgery in Kenya when no anesthetist is available: Reply. *World J Surg.* 2018 Sep;42(9):3046–3048. doi: 10.1007/s00268-018-4521-1

3. Cheng D, Barreiro G, Khan F, Mellin-Olsen J. Commentary on Burke TF et al., Safety and feasibility of a ketamine package to support emergency and essential surgery in Kenya when no anesthetist is available: An analysis of 1216 consecutive operative procedures. *World J Surg.* 2018 Sep;42(9):3042–3043. doi: 10.1007/s00268-017-4456-y

4. Litswa L. Safety and feasibility of a ketamine package to support emergency and essential surgery in Kenya when no anaesthetist is available. *World J Surg.* 2018 Sep;42(9):3044–3045. doi: 10.1007/s00268-017-4458-9

5. Burke TF, Nelson BD, Kandler T, et al. Evaluation of a ketamine-based anesthesia package for use in emergency cesarean delivery or emergency laparotomy when no anesthetist is available. *Int J Gynaecol Obstet.* 2016 Dec;135(3):295–298. doi: 10.1016/j.ijgo.2016.06.024

6. Masaki CO, Makin J, Suarez S, et al. Feasibility of a ketamine anesthesia package in support of obstetric and gynecologic procedures in Kenya when no anesthetist is available. *Afr J Reprod Health.* 2019 Mar;23(1):37–45. doi: 10.29063/ajrh2019/v23i1.4.

7. Gilder ME, Tun NW, Carter A, et al. Outcomes for 298 breastfed neonates whose mothers received ketamine and diazepam for postpartum tubal ligation in a resource-limited setting. *BMC Pregnancy Childbirth*. 2021 Feb 9;21(1):121. doi: 10.1186/s12884-021-03610-1

8. Villegas S, Suarez S, Owuor J, et al. Intraoperative awareness and experience with a ketamine-based anaesthesia package to support emergency and essential surgery when no anaesthetist is available. *Afr J Emerg Med*. 2019;9(Suppl):S56–S60. doi: 10.1016/j.afjem.2018.07.003

49

Do Checklists Improve Surgical Outcomes in Under-Resourced Settings?

PRIYANSH SHAH, MONALI MOHAN, ANITA GADGIL, AND NOBHOJIT ROY

Introduction of the WHO Surgical Safety Checklist into operating rooms in eight diverse hospitals was associated with marked improvements in surgical outcomes.
—SAFE SURGERY SAVES LIVES STUDY GROUP[1]

Research Question: Does a Surgical Safety Checklist (SSCL) reduce complications and deaths associated with surgery in high-income countries (HICs) and low- and middle-income countries (LMICs)?

Funding: Grants from the World Health Organization (WHO)

Year Study Began: 2007

Year Study Published: 2009

Study Location: 8 hospitals in 8 cities (Toronto, Canada; New Delhi, India; Amman, Jordan; Auckland, New Zealand; Manila, Philippines; Ifakara, Tanzania; London, UK; and Seattle, Washington, USA).

Who Was Studied: Consecutively enrolled patients 16 years of age or older who underwent noncardiac surgery before vs. after implementation of the SSCL.

Who Was Excluded: Patients under the age of 16 years and those who underwent cardiac surgeries.

How Many Patients Overall: 7688 patients

Study Overview: See Figure 49.1.

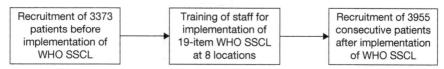

Figure 49.1. Overview of the study design.

Study Intervention: The SSCL was integrated into surgical care in 2 steps. The first step encompassed provision of information about areas of deficiencies to each local investigator. This was followed by implementing the 19-item WHO SSCL after training.

The authors conducted a prospective study of pre-intervention and post-intervention periods during which data about 6 safety indicators were collected. These 6 indicators included performance of objective airway evaluation, pulse oximeter usage, establishing 2 IV cannulas when blood loss >500 cc was expected, prophylactic antibiotics administration, oral confirmation of patient's identity and surgery site, and completion of sponge count.

Follow-Up: Discharge or 30 days after the operation

Endpoints:
> Primary outcomes: postoperative deaths and any complication; improvement in the 6 safety measures mentioned above was also accessed.

RESULTS

- Overall deaths dropped by 47% and complications by 36% after introduction of the checklist. This difference was mostly attributable to improvements in LMICs.
- The overall rates of surgical-site infection declined from 6.2% to 3.4% (p <0.001). This difference was mostly attributable to improvements in LMICs.
- The measurement of all 6 safety indicators improved by 22.5% after checklist implementation (Table 49.1).

Table 49.1 Comparison of Outcome Variations in High-Income and Low- and Middle-Income Countries

Parameter	Overall		p value	High-Income Countries		p Value	Low- and Middle-Income Countries		p value
	Before intervention	After intervention		Before intervention	After intervention		Before intervention	After intervention	
Death	1.5%	0.8%	0.003	0.9%	0.6%	0.18	2.1%	1.0%	0.006
Complications	11.0%	7.0%	<0.001	10.3%	7.1%	<0.001	11.7%	6.8%	<0.001

Criticisms and Limitations: The primary limitation of this study is that it was a simple pre- and post-analysis without a contemporaneous control group; thus the findings may have been confounded by other changes that occurred during the study period. In addition, the checklist tool was implemented under the supervision of a full-time paid supervisor, which is not feasible in many resource-constrained locations.

Other Relevant Studies and Information:

- Several other studies have demonstrated the effectiveness of surgical checklists for reducing complication rates.[2-4] There have been a push toward improving team dynamics among all levels of the healthcare team and a shift in hospital culture toward patient safety which have been widely discussed.[5,6]
- Other large analyses have failed to demonstrate clear benefits of SSCLs.[1,7]
- Despite the potential benefits, adoption of SSCLs in developing settings has been inconsistent, in part due to concerns by local healthcare workers about the impact on workflow, limited access to resources and education, and failure to see the checklist as a useful tool.[4,8,9]
- Compliance rates in implementing the SSCL vary from 12% to 100%, as documented in multiple systematic reviews, and further study may help elucidate barriers to implementation.[4,10,11]

Summary and Implications: Implementation of the SSCL reduces the overall surgical mortality rate, complication rate, and overall rates of surgical site infection, largely attributable to improvements in outcomes in LMICs.

CLINICAL CASE: CONSIDERATIONS FOR STAFF BUY-IN FOR IMPLEMENTATION OF A SURGICAL SAFETY CHECKLIST

Case History

You are a surgeon at a district hospital in a resource-constrained setting. You have recently read about the SSCL and are not completely convinced about extrapolating its use to your operating theater. You decide to discuss it with the operating theater technician, whose job includes both managing the operating theater logistics as well as providing anesthesia. What kinds of concerns do you think the operating theater technician would have on seeing the checklist elements?

Suggested Answer

Based on the discussion above, the operating theater technician in a resource-denied setting may challenge the benefit of most of the elements in the checklist. They and your other team members may benefit from discussion, explanation, and tailoring of the checklist to fit your hospital and operating theater.

For example, one of the elements mentions "The pulse oximeter is on the patient and functioning." The technician may bring up his concern that if a pulse oximeter is not working and there are no replacements or batteries in stock, it may take months to replace that item and re-establish the supply chain. This could result in the delay of surgery for an inordinate amount of time. As surgeries in the queue continue to get postponed, transferred, or canceled, this could lead to excessive out-of-pocket expenditure (travel, supplies, extra food, etc.) for the patients.

In many real-life scenarios in similar settings, the answer is not straightforward. To make this checklist contextually relevant and truly global, the local culture of the operating theater needs to be incorporated. For this case scenario, one possible solution would be to discuss the importance of having a functioning pulse oximeter with the operation theater technician for every surgery and adding assessment of the pulse oximeter instrument, along with keeping a replacement unit, as a part of the daily routine. Additionally, in case the pulse oximeter is not available/faulty, a pre-discussed consensual plan among the healthcare team and the hospital management team, regarding whether to proceed with the surgery or not, could be set in place. This would help transfer the responsibility of decision-making from one person to the team, potentially improving compliance toward checklist usage.

References

1. Haynes AB, Weiser TG, Berry WR, et al.; Safe Surgery Saves Lives Study Group. A surgical safety checklist to reduce morbidity and mortality in a global population. *N Engl J Med.* 2009 Jan 29;360(5):491–499. doi: 10.1056/NEJMsa0810119. PMID: 19144931.
2. Abbott TEF, Ahmad T, Phull MK, et al. The surgical safety checklist and patient outcomes after surgery: A prospective observational cohort study, systematic review and meta-analysis. *Br J Anaesth.* 2018;120:146–155.

3. Lau CSM, Chamberlain RS. The World Health Organization Surgical Safety Checklist Improves post-operative outcomes: A meta-analysis and systematic review. *Surg Sci.* 2016;7:206–217.

4. Treadwell JR, Lucas S, Tsou AY. Surgical checklists: A systematic review of impacts and implementation. *BMJ Qual Saf.* 2014 Apr;23(4):299–318. doi: 10.1136/bmjqs-2012-001797. PMID: 23922403; PMCID: PMC3963558.

5. Russ S, Rout S, Sevdalis N, Moorthy K, Darzi A, Vincent C. Do safety checklists improve teamwork and communication in the operating room? A systematic review. *Ann Surg.* 2013;258:856–871.

6. Sacks GD, Shannon EM, Dawes AJ, et al. Teamwork, communication and safety climate: A systematic review of interventions to improve surgical culture. *BMJ Qual Saf.* 2015;24:458–467.

7. Urbach D, Govindarajan A, Saskin R, Wilton A, Baxter N. Adoption of surgical safety checklists in Ontario, Canada: Overpromised or underdelivered? *Healthc Q.* 2014;17:10–12.

8. Epiu I, Tindimwebwa JV, Mijumbi C, et al. Working towards safer surgery in Africa; a survey of utilization of the WHO safe surgical checklist at the main referral hospitals in East Africa. *BMC Anesthesiol.* 2016;16(1):60. Published 2016 Aug 11. doi: 10.1186/s12871-016-0228-8

9. Tostes MF do P, Galvão CM. Implementation process of the Surgical Safety Checklist: Integrative review. *Rev Lat Am Enfermagem.* 2019;27:

10. Bergs J, Hellings J, Cleemput Z, et al. Systematic review and meta-analysis of the effect of the World Health Organization surgical safety checklist on postoperative complications. *Br J Surg.* 2014;101(3):150–158.

11. Borchard A, Schwappach DL, Barbir A, Bezzola P. A systematic review of the effectiveness, compliance, and critical factors for implementation of safety checklists in surgery. *Ann Surg.* 2012 Dec;256(6):925–933. doi: 10.1097/SLA.0b013e3182682f27. PMID: 22968074.

50

Task-Shifting for Caesarean Section

Can Clinical Officers Provide Equivalent Quality of Care Where There Are No Doctors?

SITALIRE KAPIRA AND MARIA OPENSHAW

Enhanced access to emergency obstetric surgery through greater deployment of clinical officers, in countries with poor coverage by doctors, can form part of the solution to meet Millennium Development Goals.[1]

Research Question: Are clinical officers (COs; nonphysician clinicians trained to perform tasks traditionally undertaken by physicians) as safe and effective as medical doctors (MDs) when performing caesarean sections in developing countries?

Funding: Ammalife, Birmingham Women's NHS foundation Trust R&D Department

Year Study Began: Meta-analysis of studies published during 1987–2009

Year Study Published: 2011

Study Location: Zaire, Malawi, Tanzania, Mozambique, Burkina Faso

Who Was Studied: This study was a systematic review and meta-analysis of 6 non-randomized controlled trials comparing the surgical outcomes of clinical officers and medical doctors performing caesarean sections in developing countries.

Who Was Excluded: Any study that was not controlled, did not compare clinical officers with medically trained doctors, or did not report on clinically relevant maternal or perinatal outcomes.

How Many Patients: 16 018

Study Overview: See Figure 50.1.

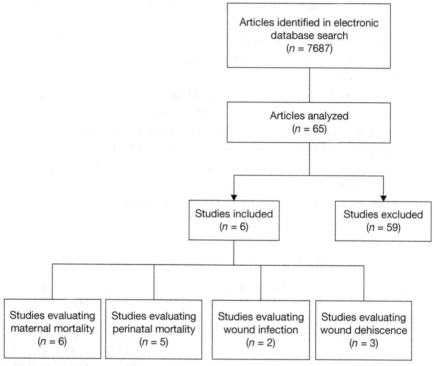

Figure 50.1. Summary of the study.

Study Intervention: Six studies were selected for inclusion by two reviewers. Tables were created with information on study characteristics, quality, and outcome data, as well as review of descriptive information on the role of the clinical officer. The Newcastle-Ottawa scale was used to evaluate selected studies for methodological quality, including selection, comparability, and outcome measures. Then, the random effects model was used to pool the odds ratios from individual studies. Heterogeneity was evaluated using forest plots and chi-square tests.

Follow-Up: Since the data were collected retrospectively, no follow-up was conducted.

Endpoints: Maternal mortality, perinatal mortality, wound infection, and wound dehiscence.

RESULTS

- The overall maternal mortality ratio was high in all 6 studies at 1211 per 100 000 live births compared to a reported 462 per 100 000 live births in low-income countries and 11 per 100 000 live births in HIC according to the WHO (Table 50.1).[2]
- There were no statistically significant differences in maternal or perinatal mortality overall between patients who were cared for by COs or MDs.
- Patients treated by COs were statistically more likely to have wound dehiscence or wound infection complications.
- Some of the included studies initially showed increased maternal and neonatal mortality for surgeries performed by COs vs. physicians; however, upon adjustment for confounders done in the original studies these differences were not statistically significant. There was no heterogeneity among studies for wound infection and dehiscence.

Table 50.1 SUMMARY OF THE META-ANALYSIS

Outcome	Complication Rates		*p* Value	Odds Ratio (95% CI)
	Clinical Officer	Medical Doctor		
Maternal Mortality	1.4%	0.9%	0.24	1.46 (0.78–2.75)
Perinatal Mortality	11.7%	7.7%	0.19	1.31 (0.78–1.95)
Wound Infection	5.8%	1.5%	0.05	1.58 (1.01–2.47)
Wound Dehiscence	2.6%	0.6%	0.005	1.89 (1.21–2.95)

Criticisms and Limitations:

- Generalizability is limited as the included studies spanned a 20-year period, 5 African countries, and diversity in clinical training program length and quality, geography, and practice settings.
- The lack of randomization may have resulted in bias as more complex or emergency procedures may have been more likely to go to either MDs or COs depending on the clinical setting, which may have confounded the results.

Other Relevant Studies and Information:

- When compared with doctors, nonphysician clinicians cost less to train and employ, generally require shorter training periods, and are noted to be the "backbone" of healthcare in many areas and specialties where there are physician shortages. Studies demonstrate that task-shifting can reduce morbidity and mortality and reduce health disparities in care delivery.[3–6] Despite evidence that task-shifting can be an effective way to improve health equity, there are barriers to its implementation. These include resistant attitudes toward task-shifting and regulatory/professional issues.[7]
- Studies published in the years since publication of this review have focused on evaluation of surgical training for COs to enhance skill acquisition as well as emergency obstetric skills.[8–10]

Summary and Implications: This review suggests that care provided by COs and physicians for women and neonates undergoing caesarean section are associated with similar mortality rates, though care from COs may be associated with higher rates of complications. Since this was not a randomized trial, however, the findings are not definitive. Nevertheless, future research should focus on maximizing the safety of procedures performed by COs in situations in which no physician is available.

CLINICAL CASE: TASK SHIFTING AND ACCESS TO CARE

Case History

A 17-year-old Gravida 1 Para 0 is brought to the health center in the second stage of labor after failing to deliver at home. The nurse immediately refers her to a district hospital which is 42 km away from the health center on a muddy road. The ambulance takes 1 hour to arrive and another 45 minutes to reach the district hospital. There, the woman is seen by the CO on call who notices that the fetal heart tones are below normal. There are only 2 physicians in the entire district and they are each dealing with separate emergencies in other wards. The patient is taken to the operating theater by the CO for an emergency cesarean section and neonatal resuscitation is initiated.

1. Would the clinical outcomes have differed if a medical doctor had been available to operate?

2. What social, clinical, and health systems factors may affect this patient's ability to receive timely and appropriate care?

Suggested Answer

In this case, the fetus would likely have died in the absence of intervention. Furthermore, obstructed labor may have led to the death of the mother. In an emergency situation, the ability of a CO trained in cesarean section may have saved this baby's life as well as the mother's.

Many factors affect this patient's access to care. She lives far from a hospital with operative capability and had to be transferred for appropriate care. The unpaved roads make transport challenging. While the nurse at the rural health center made a quick assessment, the health system responded slowly and her referral and subsequent surgical intervention were delayed due to transportation and systems factors. The high clinical burden on a sparse team of physicians may have meant her care would be further delayed, had not a trained CO been present to perform her surgery. However, task-shifting enabled her to eventually get the care she needed once she arrived at the district hospital.

References

1. Wilson A, Lissauer D, Thangaratinam S, Khan KS, MacArthur C, Coomarasamy A. A comparison of clinical officers with medical doctors on outcomes of caesarean section in the developing world: meta-analysis of controlled studies. *BMJ*. 2011;342:d2600. https://doi.org/10.1136/bmj.d2600

2. Maternal mortality. World Health Organization; September 19, 2019. Accessed October 26, 2021. https://www.who.int/news-room/fact-sheets/detail/maternal-mortality

3. Joshi R, Alim M, Kengne AP, et al. Task shifting for non-communicable disease management in low and middle income countries: A systematic review. *PLoS One*. 2014;9:e103754.

4. Kim K, Choi JS, Choi E, et al. Effects of community-based health worker interventions to improve chronic disease management and care among vulnerable populations: A systematic review. *Am J Public Health*. 2016;106(4):E3–E28.

5. Kredo T, Adeniyi FB, Bateganya M, Pienaar ED. Task shifting from doctors to non-doctors for initiation and maintenance of antiretroviral therapy. *Cochrane Database Syst Rev*. 2014 Jul 1;(7):CD007331. doi: 10.1002/14651858.CD007331.pub3. PMID: 24980859.

6. Lewin S, Munabi-Babigumira S, Glenton C, et al. Lay health workers in primary and community health care for maternal and child health and the management of infectious diseases. *Cochrane Database Syst Rev*. 2010;3:CD004015.

7. van Heemskerken P, Broekhuizen H, Gajewski J, Brugha R, Bijlmakers L. Barriers to surgery performed by non-physician clinicians in sub-Saharan Africa: A scoping review. *Human Res Health*. 2020;18(1):51. https://doi.org/10.1186/s12960-020-00490-y

8. Ellard DR, Chimwaza W, Davies D, et al.; on behalf of The ETATMBA Study Group. Can training in advanced clinical skills in obstetrics, neonatal care and leadership, of non-physician clinicians in Malawi impact on clinical services improvements (the ETATMBA project): A process evaluation. *BMJ Open.* 2014;4(8):e005751– e005751. https://doi.org/10.1136/bmjopen-2014-005751

9. Gajewski J, Borgstein E, Bijlmakers L, et al. Evaluation of a surgical training programme for clinical officers in Malawi. *Br J Surg.* 2019;106(2):e156–e165. https://doi.org/10.1002/bjs.11065

10. Liu B, Hunt LM, Lonsdale RJ, et al. Comparison of surgical skill acquisition by UK surgical trainees and Sierra Leonean associate clinicians in a task-sharing programme. *BJS Open.* 2019;3(2):218–223. https://doi.org/10.1002/bjs5.50122

INDEX